COHN-S Exam

SECRETS

Study Guide

Your Key to Exam Success

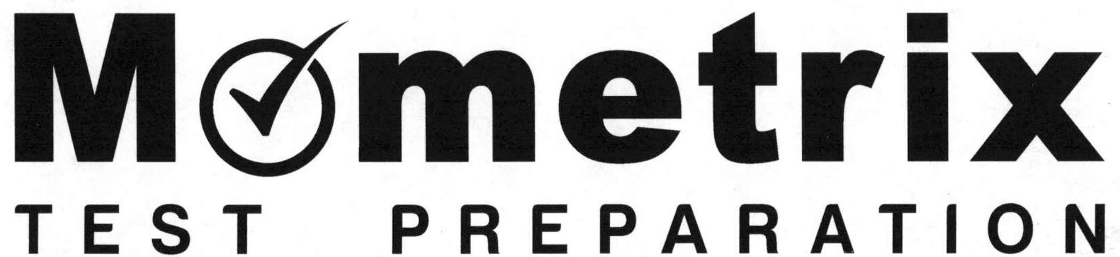

Dear Future Exam Success Story

First of all, **THANK YOU** for purchasing Mometrix study materials!

Second, congratulations! You are one of the few determined test-takers who are committed to doing whatever it takes to excel on your exam. **You have come to the right place.** We developed these study materials with one goal in mind: to deliver you the information you need in a format that's concise and easy to use.

In addition to optimizing your guide for the content of the test, we've outlined our recommended steps for breaking down the preparation process into small, attainable goals so you can make sure you stay on track.

We've also analyzed the entire test-taking process, identifying the most common pitfalls and showing how you can overcome them and be ready for any curveball the test throws you.

Standardized testing is one of the biggest obstacles on your road to success, which only increases the importance of doing well in the high-pressure, high-stakes environment of test day. Your results on this test could have a significant impact on your future, and this guide provides the information and practical advice to help you achieve your full potential on test day.

Your success is our success

We would love to hear from you! If you would like to share the story of your exam success or if you have any questions or comments in regard to our products, please contact us at **800-673-8175** or **support@mometrix.com**.

Thanks again for your business and we wish you continued success!

Sincerely,
The Mometrix Test Preparation Team

Need more help? Check out our flashcards at:
http://mometrixflashcards.com/COHN

Written and edited by the Mometrix Exam Secrets Test Prep Team
Printed in the United States of America

TABLE OF CONTENTS

Introduction

Thank you for purchasing this resource! You have made the choice to prepare yourself for a test that could have a huge impact on your future, and this guide is designed to help you be fully ready for test day. Obviously, it's important to have a solid understanding of the test material, but you also need to be prepared for the unique environment and stressors of the test, so that you can perform to the best of your abilities.

For this purpose, the first section that appears in this guide is the **Secret Keys**. We've devoted countless hours to meticulously researching what works and what doesn't, and we've boiled down our findings to the five most impactful steps you can take to improve your performance on the test. We start at the beginning with study planning and move through the preparation process, all the way to the testing strategies that will help you get the most out of what you know when you're finally sitting in front of the test.

We recommend that you start preparing for your test as far in advance as possible. However, if you've bought this guide as a last-minute study resource and only have a few days before your test, we recommend that you skip over the first two Secret Keys since they address a long-term study plan.

If you struggle with **test anxiety**, we strongly encourage you to check out our recommendations for how you can overcome it. Test anxiety is a formidable foe, but it can be beaten, and we want to make sure you have the tools you need to defeat it.

Secret Key #1 – Plan Big, Study Small

There's a lot riding on your performance. If you want to ace this test, you're going to need to keep your skills sharp and the material fresh in your mind. You need a plan that lets you review everything you need to know while still fitting in your schedule. We'll break this strategy down into three categories.

Information Organization

Start with the information you already have: the official test outline. From this, you can make a complete list of all the concepts you need to cover before the test. Organize these concepts into groups that can be studied together, and create a list of any related vocabulary you need to learn so you can brush up on any difficult terms. You'll want to keep this vocabulary list handy once you actually start studying since you may need to add to it along the way.

Time Management

Once you have your set of study concepts, decide how to spread them out over the time you have left before the test. Break your study plan into small, clear goals so you have a manageable task for each day and know exactly what you're doing. Then just focus on one small step at a time. When you manage your time this way, you don't need to spend hours at a time studying. Studying a small block of content for a short period each day helps you retain information better and avoid stressing over how much you have left to do. You can relax knowing that you have a plan to cover everything in time. In order for this strategy to be effective though, you have to start studying early and stick to your schedule. Avoid the exhaustion and futility that comes from last-minute cramming!

Study Environment

The environment you study in has a big impact on your learning. Studying in a coffee shop, while probably more enjoyable, is not likely to be as fruitful as studying in a quiet room. It's important to keep distractions to a minimum. You're only planning to study for a short block of time, so make the most of it. Don't pause to check your phone or get up to find a snack. It's also important to **avoid multitasking**. Research has consistently shown that multitasking will make your studying dramatically less effective. Your study area should also be comfortable and well-lit so you don't have the distraction of straining your eyes or sitting on an uncomfortable chair.

The time of day you study is also important. You want to be rested and alert. Don't wait until just before bedtime. Study when you'll be most likely to comprehend and remember. Even better, if you know what time of day your test will be, set that time aside for study. That way your brain will be used to working on that subject at that specific time and you'll have a better chance of recalling information.

Finally, it can be helpful to team up with others who are studying for the same test. Your actual studying should be done in as isolated an environment as possible, but the work of organizing the information and setting up the study plan can be divided up. In between study sessions, you can discuss with your teammates the concepts that you're all studying and quiz each other on the details. Just be sure that your teammates are as serious about the test as you are. If you find that your study time is being replaced with social time, you might need to find a new team.

Secret Key #2 – Make Your Studying Count

You're devoting a lot of time and effort to preparing for this test, so you want to be absolutely certain it will pay off. This means doing more than just reading the content and hoping you can remember it on test day. It's important to make every minute of study count. There are two main areas you can focus on to make your studying count:

Retention

It doesn't matter how much time you study if you can't remember the material. You need to make sure you are retaining the concepts. To check your retention of the information you're learning, try recalling it at later times with minimal prompting. Try carrying around flashcards and glance at one or two from time to time or ask a friend who's also studying for the test to quiz you.

To enhance your retention, look for ways to put the information into practice so that you can apply it rather than simply recalling it. If you're using the information in practical ways, it will be much easier to remember. Similarly, it helps to solidify a concept in your mind if you're not only reading it to yourself but also explaining it to someone else. Ask a friend to let you teach them about a concept you're a little shaky on (or speak aloud to an imaginary audience if necessary). As you try to summarize, define, give examples, and answer your friend's questions, you'll understand the concepts better and they will stay with you longer. Finally, step back for a big picture view and ask yourself how each piece of information fits with the whole subject. When you link the different concepts together and see them working together as a whole, it's easier to remember the individual components.

Finally, practice showing your work on any multi-step problems, even if you're just studying. Writing out each step you take to solve a problem will help solidify the process in your mind, and you'll be more likely to remember it during the test.

Modality

Modality simply refers to the means or method by which you study. Choosing a study modality that fits your own individual learning style is crucial. No two people learn best in exactly the same way, so it's important to know your strengths and use them to your advantage.

For example, if you learn best by visualization, focus on visualizing a concept in your mind and draw an image or a diagram. Try color-coding your notes, illustrating them, or creating symbols that will trigger your mind to recall a learned concept. If you learn best by hearing or discussing information, find a study partner who learns the same way or read aloud to yourself. Think about how to put the information in your own words. Imagine that you are giving a lecture on the topic and record yourself so you can listen to it later.

For any learning style, flashcards can be helpful. Organize the information so you can take advantage of spare moments to review. Underline key words or phrases. Use different colors for different categories. Mnemonic devices (such as creating a short list in which every item starts with the same letter) can also help with retention. Find what works best for you and use it to store the information in your mind most effectively and easily.

Secret Key #3 – Practice the Right Way

Your success on test day depends not only on how many hours you put into preparing, but also on whether you prepared the right way. It's good to check along the way to see if your studying is paying off. One of the most effective ways to do this is by taking practice tests to evaluate your progress. Practice tests are useful because they show exactly where you need to improve. Every time you take a practice test, pay special attention to these three groups of questions:

- The questions you got wrong
- The questions you had to guess on, even if you guessed right
- The questions you found difficult or slow to work through

This will show you exactly what your weak areas are, and where you need to devote more study time. Ask yourself why each of these questions gave you trouble. Was it because you didn't understand the material? Was it because you didn't remember the vocabulary? Do you need more repetitions on this type of question to build speed and confidence? Dig into those questions and figure out how you can strengthen your weak areas as you go back to review the material.

Additionally, many practice tests have a section explaining the answer choices. It can be tempting to read the explanation and think that you now have a good understanding of the concept. However, an explanation likely only covers part of the question's broader context. Even if the explanation makes sense, **go back and investigate** every concept related to the question until you're positive you have a thorough understanding.

As you go along, keep in mind that the practice test is just that: practice. Memorizing these questions and answers will not be very helpful on the actual test because it is unlikely to have any of the same exact questions. If you only know the right answers to the sample questions, you won't be prepared for the real thing. **Study the concepts** until you understand them fully, and then you'll be able to answer any question that shows up on the test.

It's important to wait on the practice tests until you're ready. If you take a test on your first day of study, you may be overwhelmed by the amount of material covered and how much you need to learn. Work up to it gradually.

On test day, you'll need to be prepared for answering questions, managing your time, and using the test-taking strategies you've learned. It's a lot to balance, like a mental marathon that will have a big impact on your future. Like training for a marathon, you'll need to start slowly and work your way up. When test day arrives, you'll be ready.

Start with the strategies you've read in the first two Secret Keys—plan your course and study in the way that works best for you. If you have time, consider using multiple study resources to get different approaches to the same concepts. It can be helpful to see difficult concepts from more than one angle. Then find a good source for practice tests. Many times, the test website will suggest potential study resources or provide sample tests.

Practice Test Strategy

When you're ready to start taking practice tests, follow this strategy:

Untimed and Open-Book Practice

Take the first test with no time constraints and with your notes and study guide handy. Take your time and focus on applying the strategies you've learned.

Timed and Open-Book Practice

Take the second practice test open-book as well, but set a timer and practice pacing yourself to finish in time.

Timed and Closed-Book Practice

Take any other practice tests as if it were test day. Set a timer and put away your study materials. Sit at a table or desk in a quiet room, imagine yourself at the testing center, and answer questions as quickly and accurately as possible.

Keep repeating timed and closed-book tests on a regular basis until you run out of practice tests or it's time for the actual test. Your mind will be ready for the schedule and stress of test day, and you'll be able to focus on recalling the material you've learned.

Secret Key #4 – Pace Yourself

Once you're fully prepared for the material on the test, your biggest challenge on test day will be managing your time. Just knowing that the clock is ticking can make you panic even if you have plenty of time left. Work on pacing yourself so you can build confidence against the time constraints of the exam. Pacing is a difficult skill to master, especially in a high-pressure environment, so **practice is vital**.

Set time expectations for your pace based on how much time is available. For example, if a section has 60 questions and the time limit is 30 minutes, you know you have to average 30 seconds or less per question in order to answer them all. Although 30 seconds is the hard limit, set 25 seconds per question as your goal, so you reserve extra time to spend on harder questions. When you budget extra time for the harder questions, you no longer have any reason to stress when those questions take longer to answer.

Don't let this time expectation distract you from working through the test at a calm, steady pace, but keep it in mind so you don't spend too much time on any one question. Recognize that taking extra time on one question you don't understand may keep you from answering two that you do understand later in the test. If your time limit for a question is up and you're still not sure of the answer, mark it and move on, and come back to it later if the time and the test format allow. If the testing format doesn't allow you to return to earlier questions, just make an educated guess; then put it out of your mind and move on.

On the easier questions, be careful not to rush. It may seem wise to hurry through them so you have more time for the challenging ones, but it's not worth missing one if you know the concept and just didn't take the time to read the question fully. Work efficiently but make sure you understand the question and have looked at all of the answer choices, since more than one may seem right at first.

Even if you're paying attention to the time, you may find yourself a little behind at some point. You should speed up to get back on track, but do so wisely. Don't panic; just take a few seconds less on each question until you're caught up. Don't guess without thinking, but do look through the answer choices and eliminate any you know are wrong. If you can get down to two choices, it is often worthwhile to guess from those. Once you've chosen an answer, move on and don't dwell on any that you skipped or had to hurry through. If a question was taking too long, chances are it was one of the harder ones, so you weren't as likely to get it right anyway.

On the other hand, if you find yourself getting ahead of schedule, it may be beneficial to slow down a little. The more quickly you work, the more likely you are to make a careless mistake that will affect your score. You've budgeted time for each question, so don't be afraid to spend that time. Practice an efficient but careful pace to get the most out of the time you have.

Secret Key #5 – Have a Plan for Guessing

When you're taking the test, you may find yourself stuck on a question. Some of the answer choices seem better than others, but you don't see the one answer choice that is obviously correct. What do you do?

The scenario described above is very common, yet most test takers have not effectively prepared for it. Developing and practicing a plan for guessing may be one of the single most effective uses of your time as you get ready for the exam.

In developing your plan for guessing, there are three questions to address:

- When should you start the guessing process?
- How should you narrow down the choices?
- Which answer should you choose?

When to Start the Guessing Process

Unless your plan for guessing is to select C every time (which, despite its merits, is not what we recommend), you need to leave yourself enough time to apply your answer elimination strategies. Since you have a limited amount of time for each question, that means that if you're going to give yourself the best shot at guessing correctly, you have to decide quickly whether or not you will guess.

Of course, the best-case scenario is that you don't have to guess at all, so first, see if you can answer the question based on your knowledge of the subject and basic reasoning skills. Focus on the key words in the question and try to jog your memory of related topics. Give yourself a chance to bring the knowledge to mind, but once you realize that you don't have (or you can't access) the knowledge you need to answer the question, it's time to start the guessing process.

It's almost always better to start the guessing process too early than too late. It only takes a few seconds to remember something and answer the question from knowledge. Carefully eliminating wrong answer choices takes longer. Plus, going through the process of eliminating answer choices can actually help jog your memory.

Summary: Start the guessing process as soon as you decide that you can't answer the question based on your knowledge.

How to Narrow Down the Choices

The next chapter in this book (**Test-Taking Strategies**) includes a wide range of strategies for how to approach questions and how to look for answer choices to eliminate. You will definitely want to read those carefully, practice them, and figure out which ones work best for you. Here though, we're going to address a mindset rather than a particular strategy.

Your chances of guessing an answer correctly depend on how many options you are choosing from.

How many choices you have	How likely you are to guess correctly
5	20%
4	25%
3	33%
2	50%
1	100%

You can see from this chart just how valuable it is to be able to eliminate incorrect answers and make an educated guess, but there are two things that many test takers do that cause them to miss out on the benefits of guessing:

- Accidentally eliminating the correct answer
- Selecting an answer based on an impression

We'll look at the first one here, and the second one in the next section.

To avoid accidentally eliminating the correct answer, we recommend a thought exercise called **the $5 challenge**. In this challenge, you only eliminate an answer choice from contention if you are willing to bet $5 on it being wrong. Why $5? Five dollars is a small but not insignificant amount of money. It's an amount you could afford to lose but wouldn't want to throw away. And while losing $5 once might not hurt too much, doing it twenty times will set you back $100. In the same way, each small decision you make—eliminating a choice here, guessing on a question there—won't by itself impact your score very much, but when you put them all together, they can make a big difference. By holding each answer choice elimination decision to a higher standard, you can reduce the risk of accidentally eliminating the correct answer.

The $5 challenge can also be applied in a positive sense: If you are willing to bet $5 that an answer choice *is* correct, go ahead and mark it as correct.

Summary: Only eliminate an answer choice if you are willing to bet $5 that it is wrong.

Which Answer to Choose

You're taking the test. You've run into a hard question and decided you'll have to guess. You've eliminated all the answer choices you're willing to bet $5 on. Now you have to pick an answer. Why do we even need to talk about this? Why can't you just pick whichever one you feel like when the time comes?

The answer to these questions is that if you don't come into the test with a plan, you'll rely on your impression to select an answer choice, and if you do that, you risk falling into a trap. The test writers know that everyone who takes their test will be guessing on some of the questions, so they intentionally write wrong answer choices to seem plausible. You still have to pick an answer though, and if the wrong answer choices are designed to look right, how can you ever be sure that you're not falling for their trap? The best solution we've found to this dilemma is to take the decision out of your hands entirely. Here is the process we recommend:

Once you've eliminated any choices that you are confident (willing to bet $5) are wrong, select the first remaining choice as your answer.

Whether you choose to select the first remaining choice, the second, or the last, the important thing is that you use some preselected standard. Using this approach guarantees that you will not be enticed into selecting an answer choice that looks right, because you are not basing your decision on how the answer choices look.

This is not meant to make you question your knowledge. Instead, it is to help you recognize the difference between your knowledge and your impressions. There's a huge difference between thinking an answer is right because of what you know, and thinking an answer is right because it looks or sounds like it should be right.

Summary: To ensure that your selection is appropriately random, make a predetermined selection from among all answer choices you have not eliminated.

Test-Taking Strategies

This section contains a list of test-taking strategies that you may find helpful as you work through the test. By taking what you know and applying logical thought, you can maximize your chances of answering any question correctly!

It is very important to realize that every question is different and every person is different: no single strategy will work on every question, and no single strategy will work for every person. That's why we've included all of them here, so you can try them out and determine which ones work best for different types of questions and which ones work best for you.

Question Strategies

Read Carefully

Read the question and answer choices carefully. Don't miss the question because you misread the terms. You have plenty of time to read each question thoroughly and make sure you understand what is being asked. Yet a happy medium must be attained, so don't waste too much time. You must read carefully, but efficiently.

Contextual Clues

Look for contextual clues. If the question includes a word you are not familiar with, look at the immediate context for some indication of what the word might mean. Contextual clues can often give you all the information you need to decipher the meaning of an unfamiliar word. Even if you can't determine the meaning, you may be able to narrow down the possibilities enough to make a solid guess at the answer to the question.

Prefixes

If you're having trouble with a word in the question or answer choices, try dissecting it. Take advantage of every clue that the word might include. Prefixes and suffixes can be a huge help. Usually they allow you to determine a basic meaning. Pre- means before, post- means after, pro - is positive, de- is negative. From prefixes and suffixes, you can get an idea of the general meaning of the word and try to put it into context.

Hedge Words

Watch out for critical hedge words, such as *likely, may, can, sometimes, often, almost, mostly, usually, generally, rarely,* and *sometimes.* Question writers insert these hedge phrases to cover every possibility. Often an answer choice will be wrong simply because it leaves no room for exception. Be on guard for answer choices that have definitive words such as *exactly* and *always.*

Switchback Words

Stay alert for *switchbacks.* These are the words and phrases frequently used to alert you to shifts in thought. The most common switchback words are *but, although,* and *however.* Others include *nevertheless, on the other hand, even though, while, in spite of, despite, regardless of.* Switchback words are important to catch because they can change the direction of the question or an answer choice.

FACE VALUE

When in doubt, use common sense. Accept the situation in the problem at face value. Don't read too much into it. These problems will not require you to make wild assumptions. If you have to go beyond creativity and warp time or space in order to have an answer choice fit the question, then you should move on and consider the other answer choices. These are normal problems rooted in reality. The applicable relationship or explanation may not be readily apparent, but it is there for you to figure out. Use your common sense to interpret anything that isn't clear.

Answer Choice Strategies

ANSWER SELECTION

The most thorough way to pick an answer choice is to identify and eliminate wrong answers until only one is left, then confirm it is the correct answer. Sometimes an answer choice may immediately seem right, but be careful. The test writers will usually put more than one reasonable answer choice on each question, so take a second to read all of them and make sure that the other choices are not equally obvious. As long as you have time left, it is better to read every answer choice than to pick the first one that looks right without checking the others.

ANSWER CHOICE FAMILIES

An answer choice family consists of two (in rare cases, three) answer choices that are very similar in construction and cannot all be true at the same time. If you see two answer choices that are direct opposites or parallels, one of them is usually the correct answer. For instance, if one answer choice says that quantity *x* increases and another either says that quantity *x* decreases (opposite) or says that quantity *y* increases (parallel), then those answer choices would fall into the same family. An answer choice that doesn't match the construction of the answer choice family is more likely to be incorrect. Most questions will not have answer choice families, but when they do appear, you should be prepared to recognize them.

ELIMINATE ANSWERS

Eliminate answer choices as soon as you realize they are wrong, but make sure you consider all possibilities. If you are eliminating answer choices and realize that the last one you are left with is also wrong, don't panic. Start over and consider each choice again. There may be something you missed the first time that you will realize on the second pass.

AVOID FACT TRAPS

Don't be distracted by an answer choice that is factually true but doesn't answer the question. You are looking for the choice that answers the question. Stay focused on what the question is asking for so you don't accidentally pick an answer that is true but incorrect. Always go back to the question and make sure the answer choice you've selected actually answers the question and is not merely a true statement.

EXTREME STATEMENTS

In general, you should avoid answers that put forth extreme actions as standard practice or proclaim controversial ideas as established fact. An answer choice that states the "process should be used in certain situations, if…" is much more likely to be correct than one that states the "process should be discontinued completely." The first is a calm rational statement and doesn't even make a definitive, uncompromising stance, using a hedge word *if* to provide wiggle room, whereas the second choice is a radical idea and far more extreme.

Benchmark

As you read through the answer choices and you come across one that seems to answer the question well, mentally select that answer choice. This is not your final answer, but it's the one that will help you evaluate the other answer choices. The one that you selected is your benchmark or standard for judging each of the other answer choices. Every other answer choice must be compared to your benchmark. That choice is correct until proven otherwise by another answer choice beating it. If you find a better answer, then that one becomes your new benchmark. Once you've decided that no other choice answers the question as well as your benchmark, you have your final answer.

Predict the Answer

Before you even start looking at the answer choices, it is often best to try to predict the answer. When you come up with the answer on your own, it is easier to avoid distractions and traps because you will know exactly what to look for. The right answer choice is unlikely to be word-for-word what you came up with, but it should be a close match. Even if you are confident that you have the right answer, you should still take the time to read each option before moving on.

General Strategies

Tough Questions

If you are stumped on a problem or it appears too hard or too difficult, don't waste time. Move on! Remember though, if you can quickly check for obviously incorrect answer choices, your chances of guessing correctly are greatly improved. Before you completely give up, at least try to knock out a couple of possible answers. Eliminate what you can and then guess at the remaining answer choices before moving on.

Check Your Work

Since you will probably not know every term listed and the answer to every question, it is important that you get credit for the ones that you do know. Don't miss any questions through careless mistakes. If at all possible, try to take a second to look back over your answer selection and make sure you've selected the correct answer choice and haven't made a costly careless mistake (such as marking an answer choice that you didn't mean to mark). This quick double check should more than pay for itself in caught mistakes for the time it costs.

Pace Yourself

It's easy to be overwhelmed when you're looking at a page full of questions; your mind is confused and full of random thoughts, and the clock is ticking down faster than you would like. Calm down and maintain the pace that you have set for yourself. Especially as you get down to the last few minutes of the test, don't let the small numbers on the clock make you panic. As long as you are on track by monitoring your pace, you are guaranteed to have time for each question.

Don't Rush

It is very easy to make errors when you are in a hurry. Maintaining a fast pace in answering questions is pointless if it makes you miss questions that you would have gotten right otherwise. Test writers like to include distracting information and wrong answers that seem right. Taking a little extra time to avoid careless mistakes can make all the difference in your test score. Find a pace that allows you to be confident in the answers that you select.

KEEP MOVING

Panicking will not help you pass the test, so do your best to stay calm and keep moving. Taking deep breaths and going through the answer elimination steps you practiced can help to break through a stress barrier and keep your pace.

Final Notes

The combination of a solid foundation of content knowledge and the confidence that comes from practicing your plan for applying that knowledge is the key to maximizing your performance on test day. As your foundation of content knowledge is built up and strengthened, you'll find that the strategies included in this chapter become more and more effective in helping you quickly sift through the distractions and traps of the test to isolate the correct answer.

Now it's time to move on to the test content chapters of this book, but be sure to keep your goal in mind. As you read, think about how you will be able to apply this information on the test. If you've already seen sample questions for the test and you have an idea of the question format and style, try to come up with questions of your own that you can answer based on what you're reading. This will give you valuable practice applying your knowledge in the same ways you can expect to on test day.

Good luck and good studying!

Occupational Health Nursing

Role of Occupational Health and Safety Program and Standards of Practice for COHN

An occupational health and safety program exists within the workforce for two main reasons: to improve the health of the workers and to reduce the number of work-related health risks. The **occupational health and safety nurse** plays many roles within this program. These roles are called standards of practice and are regulated by the American Association of Occupational Health Nurses (AAOHN). The AAOHN has defined 11 **standards of practice** that define competent performance in the realm of occupational health nursing. They are as follows: Assessment, diagnosis, outcome identification, planning, implementation, evaluation, resource management, professional development, collaboration, and research. The COHN fulfills many roles, to include clinician/practitioner, case manager, health promotion specialist, manager, consultant, educator, and researcher. Not only does an occupational health nurse provide medical assistance, they must also manage and organize interdisciplinary healthcare delivery in a cost-effective manner. The administrative roles of the occupational health and safety nurse are key parts of the job and they are what differentiate it from the other fields of nursing.

Roles of Occupational Health Nurse

Clinician

An occupational health nurse fulfills many roles within the workplace. In general, these roles can be divided into five categories: clinician, manager, educator, consultant, and case manager. Specifically, as a **clinician**, an occupational health nurse is responsible for making sure that employees are placed in jobs that are a fit for their skills. This entails an analysis of the requirements of a job, assessment of the abilities of the worker, on-going surveillance of individuals and groups that are in high-risk jobs, staying on top of new healthcare issues, monitoring practice-specific laws and regulations, recommending necessary changes to work process/worker placement, interpreting the results of tests, providing treatment for work related injuries, performing health-related technical tasks, maintaining health records, providing counseling services and crisis intervention, providing health promotion and education activities, complying with codes of ethics, implementing and maintaining confidentiality procedures, and evaluating the quality of care provided by occupational health services.

Manager

Specifically, as a **manager**, an occupational health nurse is responsible for monitoring and managing an occupational health and safety program. This entails assessing the organizational culture, developing program goals and objectives, developing nursing protocols, developing policies and procedures, understanding and applying management principles, implementing and coordinating health promotion and surveillance programs, implementing substance abuse programs, applying practice standards and regulations, conducting informal research, analyzing and evaluating quality and cost of services, and preparing reports for management.

Educator

Specifically, as an **educator**, an occupational health nurse is responsible for meeting the health and safety education/training needs of the workforce. This entails conducting an education/training needs assessment, developing plans and strategies for delivering health and safety information, developing learner objectives, planning and implementing education/training programs, evaluating the content and outcomes of education/training programs, and reporting the results of program evaluation.

Consultant

Specifically, as a **consultant**, an occupational health nurse is responsible for organizing and implementing basic health and safety programs. This entails assessing health and safety needs, conducting job analyses and worksite walk-through assessments, investigated environmental health issues, developing and implementing hazard remediation plans, reviewing SDS's and recommending appropriate hazard control measures, providing necessary information and resources, and evaluating data and controls to determine program efficacy.

Case Manager

Specifically, as a **case manager**, an occupational health nurse is responsible for establishing and implementing case management protocols. This entails identifying cases that require case management; developing and managing case management plans and programs; developing a multidisciplinary approach to case management that includes building a network of resources; disability program administration (STD, LTD, FMLA, workers comp, ADA); risk management program management; evaluating quality of care; assessing outcomes of care as compared to treatment plans; and staying on top of the legal, labor, and regulatory aspects of case management.

Workplace Hazards

Assessment

Workplace Hazards

Hazards within the workplace can be divided into **five different categories.** They are as follows:

- **Biological/Infection Hazards**: Biological agents (bacteria, viruses, fungi) that can be transmitted from one person to another.
- **Chemical Hazards**: Chemicals that have are potentially toxic (including medications, solutions, gases, vapors, aerosols, particulate matter).
- **Environmental Hazards**: Factors within the workplace that can cause injuries, strain, or discomfort.
- **Physical Hazards**: Aspects of the work environment (such as radiation, electricity, temperature, and noise) that can cause physical harm.
- **Psychosocial Hazards**: Aspects of the job or work environment that can cause emotional stress, strain, or interpersonal problems.

Identification

The success of any occupational health program depends greatly on the occupational health nurse's ability to understand and identify hazards in the workplace. The **identification of workplace hazards** entails a process of assessing the work environment, and this is done primarily by walking through the worksite (walk-throughs). It is often the case that the occupational health nurse is the only licensed professional at the worksite, and so plays a crucial role in the assessment process. Not only does the nurse need to have a solid understanding of occupational health science, they need to be familiar with the all of the different aspects of the work environment (including work processes, health trends and demographics of the workforce, and workplace hazards). The goal of any assessment process is always to detect hazards and institute prevention strategies before anyone is hurt.

Multidisciplinary Approach to Occupational Healthcare

Although it is often the case that the occupational health nurse is the only licensed healthcare professional at the worksite, the most efficient and effective approach to occupational healthcare (including workplace assessment) relies on the expertise and skills of others. Thus, a multidisciplinary approach is required, incorporating the abilities of those that have knowledge specific to a particular area of occupational health and safety, including physicians, nurses, safety specialists, and industrial hygienists.

Difficulties in Assessing Frequency of Work-Related Diseases

Occupational health programs not only rely on the identification of workplace hazards, but also needs to stay on top of **the frequency of work-related diseases.** This entails an aspect of reporting and data analysis that is unique to occupational health nursing. It can be difficult, however, to obtain accurate estimates of work-related diseases for several reasons. Many problems are not brought to the attention of the occupational health office and so are not documented. It is also the case that some diseases are not recognized by the worker, supervisor, or nurse as being work-related. This is particularly the case if there is a long time between occupational exposure and the onset of symptoms.

Occupational Illnesses in Industrial Workers

Industrial workers have the largest number of occupational illnesses because they are often exposed to multiple workplace hazards as a part of doing their jobs. These risks include environmental and physical hazards; exposure to the toxic chemicals found in paints, soaps, plastics, and resins; and harmful dusts, gases, and metals. The most common occupational illnesses are musculoskeletal disorders and skin rashes. The success of any occupational health program depends greatly on the identification of workplace hazards. The identification of workplace hazards entails a process of assessing the work environment, and this is done primarily by walking through the worksite (walk-throughs).

Chemical Hazards

Toxicology

Toxicology is the study of the harmful effects that chemicals can have on organisms. Chemicals are referred to as "toxic agents" when there is harm done to an organism due to exposure. Defining toxic agents can be difficult because not all chemicals cause harm in the same dose. In fact, there are many chemicals that are considered beneficial in low doses. This is particularly the case with medicines and various medical treatment options. However, even with chemicals that have a beneficial use, if the exposure is high enough, the effect moves from beneficial to harmful, and at that point is considered toxic. Because workers come into contact with many different chemicals in the workplace, it is important to understand their potential for harmful effects. This is particularly the case in an industrial setting. The field of industrial toxicology focuses on the toxic agents in industrial settings.

Classifications of Chemicals

The American National Standards Institute

The **American National Standards Institute** defines the **five different classifications of chemicals** as follows:

1. **Dusts** - Solid particles that are the result of physical processes such as handling, crushing, grinding, rapid impact, and detonating. Dusts tend to settle on surfaces due to gravity.
2. **Fumes** - Solid particles that are the result of the condensation of gases or due to chemical reactions such as oxidations. Fumes tend to congregate as clouds in the air.
3. **Mists** - Drops of liquid that are suspended in the air due to the change of a gas to a liquid or by dispersing a liquid by splashing or foaming.
4. **Vapors** - The gaseous state of a substance that is typically found in its solid or liquid state. Vapors can be changed back to a previous state by either increasing pressure or decreasing temperature.
5. **Gases** - Fluids that tend to stay in the gaseous state, and can only be changed into a liquid or solid state by a combination of increasing pressure and decreasing temperature.

Exposure *and* Targeted Effect

In addition to classifying chemicals as dusts, fumes, mists, vapors, or gases, they can also be **classified according to the type of exposure and the targeted effect of the chemical**. Exposure is described as either acute or chronic:

- **Acute exposure** describes a high dose over a short period of time with the corresponding effect being a strong, rapid onset of symptoms with the result often being extreme damage. Acute exposure is sometimes reversible.
- **Chronic exposure** refers to small doses over a long period of time. The effect of this type of exposure does not have the rapid onset of symptoms that comes with acute exposure. The effects, however, are often irreversible.

The targeted effect of a chemical describes just how much of the body is affected by exposure. The targeted effect can be either local or systemic. **Local toxicity** has an effect restricted to the site that is exposed to the chemical, whereas a **systemic effect** has an impact on many, if not all, systems of the body.

Relationship Between Toxicity and Hazard

A chemical is considered **toxic** if it has the potential to cause harm to an organism. This harm can come in the form of damage to tissues, organs, or biochemical processes. A chemical is considered a **hazard** if the potential for damage is severe enough that is can result in poisoning. So, while both toxicity and hazard are related to toxicology, every toxic chemical is not necessarily considered a hazard. Safe work practices can eliminate or control potential hazards in the workplace. The toxicity of a substance, on the other hand, cannot be altered. It is natural part of a toxic chemical.

Health Effects of Chemical Exposure

There are three different possible **health effects due to chemical exposure**. These are mutagenic, carcinogenic, or teratogenic.

Mutagens

A **mutagenic effect** is one that results in a change (or mutation) to the DNA of an organism, and a mutagen is the substance that causes mutation. These genetic effects can be point mutations, damage to chromosomes, or interference with the mechanisms of cell division. Damage to an organism's genetic material can affect the somatic cells (non-reproductive cells in the body) or germ cells (reproductive cells such as the sperm and egg). When the damage is to germ cells, there is the potential to pass on the mutation to subsequent generations.

Carcinogens

A **carcinogenic effect** is one that causes a cell to become cancerous. Carcinogens have the potential to cause cancer through what is known as initiation and promotion. During initiation, genetic mutations occur that make the cells a potential cancer. However, because the body has ways to repair changes/damage to DNA, initiation itself does not cause cancer. It is through the process of promotion that the changes to the initiated cell are stimulated to be cancerous.

Teratogens

A **teratogenic effect** is one that involves fetal development. Teratogens can result in severe birth defects, retarded development, embryonic death, as well as postnatal learning and behavioral disorders. A fetus is extremely vulnerable to teratogens because it is in a state of development with a great deal of cell division and differentiation occurring. Just how strong the teratogenic effect is depends greatly on the age/development of the fetus, as well as dose of the chemical.

Effects of Chemical Agents on Organs/Systems

The following are chemical agents and the organs/systems that they are known to affect:

- **Aluminum**: nervous system, respiratory system
- **Arsenic**: nervous system, liver, GI tract, respiratory system, hematopoietic system, endocrine system
- **Beryllium**: respiratory system, skin
- **Bromide**: nervous system, skin
- **Cadmium**: renal system, nervous system, GI tract, respiratory system, bone, cardiovascular system
- **Chromium**: renal system, nervous system, liver, respiratory system, skin
- **Cobalt**: nervous system, GI tract, respiratory system, endocrine system, skin, cardiovascular system
- **Copper**: GI tract, hematopoietic system
- **Fluoride**: nervous system, respiratory system, bone, skin

- **Iron**: nervous system, liver, GI tract, respiratory system, hematopoietic system, endocrine system
- **Lead**: renal system, nervous system, hematopoietic system, endocrine system
- **Manganese**: nervous system, respiratory system
- **Mercury**: renal system, nervous system, GI tract, respiratory system
- **Nickel**: nervous system, respiratory system, skin
- **Selenium**: renal system, GI tract, skin
- **Silver**: respiratory system, skin
- **Thallium**: renal system, nervous system, liver, GI tract, respiratory system, bone
- **Zinc**: GI tract, hematopoietic system, bone

Harmful Properties of Chemicals

There are different ways that chemicals can be harmful, and these depend on the properties of the chemical. The **harmful properties of chemicals** include explosiveness and reactivity, flammability and combustibility, radioactivity, corrosiveness, irritation, sensitization, and toxicity. These are all natural parts of the chemical that cannot be altered. However, the degree to which any of these properties are realized depends greatly on the amount and type of chemical to which a person is exposed. Appropriate safety procedures such as proper use, safe handling, and proper storage can help reduce the potential to experience the harmful properties of any chemical.

Dose-Response, Effective Dose, and Threshold Dose Related to Chemical Toxicity

Dose-response describes the correlation between the dose of a chemical and the amount of effect that is realized. It distinguishes between doses where the response is beneficial and the dose where the response is harmful. **Effective dose** refers to the dose to which there is positive response. Effective dose applies when a chemical is used for medical treatment. In most cases, the higher the dose, the greater the response. There can, however, be a dose at which there is no effect, but after this point, the effect greatly increases. This is called the **threshold dose** and it is an important aspect of the dose-response relationship.

Latency Period

Latency period refers to the lapse in time between moment of exposure to a chemical and when an observable effect is realized. In any setting where toxic chemicals are employed, it is important to know the not just the symptoms of exposure, but the latency period for each chemical. When the latency period is short, there is a greater likelihood that the negative effects associated with the exposure with be reported to medical personnel. If the latency period is long, however, there is the possibility that when the symptoms do appear, they will not be associated with the exposure, and therefore not get reported. This results in inaccurate chemical exposure data.

Poison

A **poison** is a chemical that produces illness or death when a person is exposed to only small quantities. This designation goes a bit further than calling a chemical a toxin. A toxin is a chemical that simply produces a negative effect. All poisons are toxins, but not all toxins are poisons. The technical definition of poison is a chemical with an LD50 of 50 milligrams or less of chemical per kilogram of body weight. LD50 (lethal dose 50) refers to the amount of exposure that results in death for 50% of those exposed. The lower the LD50, the greater the level of toxicity, and the higher the LD50, the less the toxicity. Due to the inability to perform chemical tests on humans, the actual LD50 of most chemicals is unknown. However, data taken from animal experiments are interpreted and extrapolated to get an estimated lethal dose in humans.

ASPHYXIANTS

Asphyxiants are chemicals that cause a condition called hypoxia, or a decrease in the amount of oxygen available to the tissues of the body. Chemicals can cause hypoxia in several ways. Simple asphyxiants, such as carbon dioxide and nitrogen, displace the amount of oxygen in the air, resulting in a reduction in the amount of oxygen available to breath. Chemical asphyxiants block the absorption of oxygen within the body at the cellular level. Carbon monoxide is one example of a chemical asphyxiant. It causes hypoxia by binding to hemoglobin in the bloodstream, thus interfering with oxygen transport to the cells.

EXPOSURE TO CHEMICAL HAZARDS

BENZENE

Benzene (AKA benzol, carbon oil, and coal naphtha) is a non-polar (class 1B flammable liquid) substance, and exposure may result from inhalation, ingestion, and direct skin or eye contact. Exposure symptoms include:

- **Acute**: Dizziness, headache, nausea, weakness, drowsiness, altered mentation (giddiness, euphoria), GI irritation, pulmonary edema, pneumonia, skin and eye irritation, mucous membrane irritation and abdominal pain (ingestion), and CNS depression with tremors, seizures, and paralysis, and death. Acute inhalation may result in polyneuritis, CNS depression, and cardiac sensitization (life-threatening arrhythmias, ventricular fibrillation) as well as pulmonary hemorrhagic inflammation.
- **Chronic**: Nervousness, fatigue, irritability, blurred vision, difficulty breathing, skin irritation (blistering, red, dry), and scaly dermatitis. Patients may develop anorexia, aplastic anemia, and/or leukemia from damage to bone marrow.

Emergency treatment for acute exposure includes 15-minute eye flush for eye exposure, and shower and scrubbing with soap and water for skin exposure. Contaminated clothes should be double-bagged and incinerated. As there is no antidote, supportive care for pulmonary function (oxygen, intubation/mechanical ventilation) and cardiac function is indicated. For ingestion, emesis should not be induced but a slurry of activated charcoal administered if patient able to swallow. Benzodiazepine is used for seizures.

CUTTING OILS

Cutting oils are oils with additives used for cooling and lubrication in metalworking. Cutting oils often contain sulfur and/or chlorine. Some cutting oils are almost pure kerosene (which is liquid hydrocarbon derived from petroleum). WD-40 is a commonly-used cutting oil composed of fish oil and kerosene. Symptoms of exposure vary with the type of cutting oil and the route of exposure. Skin exposure may result in irritation and burns. Inhalation may cause severe respiratory irritation, and some, such as kerosene, may result in severe CNS depression (seizures, altered state of consciousness, irritability, coma, death). Emergency treatment includes skin decontamination with a shower, soap and water. Large ingestions of some hydrocarbon-containing substances (camphor, halogenated, aromatic, metal-containing, and pesticide-containing hydrocarbons), may be treated with nasogastric lavage although there are risks, such as aspiration, involved. Treatment is supportive and may include oxygen, intubation and mechanical ventilation for inhalation.

ASBESTOS

Asbestos is a group of filaments or fibers of silicates. Exposure (usually related to construction) may occur through inhalation or ingestion. Asbestos may result in lung disease (pneumoconiosis) if inhaled. Inhalation increases the risk of developing asbestosis, pulmonary cancer, and mesothelioma as well as right-sided heart failure, cor pulmonale, and pulmonary hypertension. Exposure symptoms include:

- **Acute**: May result in dyspnea and chest pain from inhalation and abdominal pain and irritation of skin and mucous membranes from ingestion.
- **Chronic**: May result in impaired pulmonary function, dyspnea, dry hacking cough, clubbing of fingers, and cyanosis of skin and mucous membranes. Disease progression is accelerated in those who smoke.

Workers coming in contact with asbestos should wear chemical protective clothing and gloves to prevent skin contact. Contaminated clothing should be removed, placed in impermeable containers, and then discarded or properly laundered. Workers should shower after work and change into clean clothing. Contaminated skin should be promptly washed with soap and water. If eyes are exposed, they should be flushed with water for 15 minutes. If exposure is necessary, then approved respirators should be used. Treatment is primarily supportive as no medications have been found to be affective.

Silica

Silica (AKA silicon dioxide [amorphous], diatomaceous earth, quartz) is a mineral and major component of sand. Inhalation of crystalline silica dust particles can result in silicosis (scar tissue forming in the lungs), a primary pneumoconiosis; and, because silica is carcinogenic, it can lead to lung cancer. High risk work includes foundry work, mining, jewelry polishing, metal grinding, stonecutting, quarry work, blasting, electric cable manufacturing, and tunneling. Prolonged or profound inhalation can result in the formation of pulmonary nodules. In early stages of silicosis, patients may be asymptomatic; but with chronic exposure, patients become increasingly dyspneic and pulmonary function obstructed and restricted. Severe progressive massive fibrosis may occur after about 5 to 10 years of exposure and can lead to respiratory failure. Silicosis increases the risk of tuberculosis, so all patients should have tuberculin skin tests and periodic chest x-rays. Risk is also increased for autoimmune diseases (rheumatoid arthritis, SLE), COPD, and chronic kidney disease. Treatment is supportive as no therapy can reverse the damage. Lung transplantation may be necessary.

Cotton Dust

Cotton dust results from processing cotton fibers along with any materials (stems, leaves, dirt) on the fibers during any phase of manufacturing, so those involved in the textile industry (yarn, fabric) are especially at risk. Exposure is through inhalation in improperly ventilated spaces. Exposure:

- **Acute/Short-term**: May result in bronchitis or acute byssinosis (brown lung disease, Monday fever), but symptoms are reversible if removed from exposure. Symptoms may include fever, chest tightening, chills, dyspnea, wheezing, weakness, and coughing.
- **Chronic**: May result in chronic byssinosis and airway obstruction with chronic bronchitis and emphysema because of permanent damage to lungs. Smoking increases risk of advanced disease.

Treatment includes eyewash station for contact with eyes. For respiratory problems, treatment may include supportive care and bronchodilators and inhaled anti-inflammatory medications mush as steroids. Treatment is similar to that for asthma. Preventive measures include improving ventilation and avoiding exposure. In some cases, respirators may be recommended.

METHANE

Methane, a component of natural gas, is colorless and odorless. People who live near or work at landfills, farms, chemical plants, wastewater treatment plants, and hydro-fracking sites are at increased risk Methane may accumulate in low-lying confined spaces. Compressed methane may explode if exposed to heat. Liquified methane may cause the skin to freeze (frostbite). Eye contact with methane gas is non-irritating, but exposure to liquid methane may cause permanent damage or blindness. Most exposure is through inhalation, and patients may lose consciousness after even one minute of exposure. If the concentration is low, the body is able to compensate, but if the concentration is high, oxygen is displaced and hypoxia can occur with altered state of consciousness, nausea, vomiting, seizures, coma and death. Emergency treatment includes:

- **Skin**: Remove patient from contamination source and remove any garments or jewelry that may restrict circulation. Follow protocols for rewarming.
- **Eye**: Gently flush eyes and cover with sterile dressing.
- **Inhalation**: Remove to area with fresh air and provide oxygen as needed. Some may require intubation and mechanical ventilation.

CYANIDE

Cyanide, a poisonous chemical containing a carbon-nitrogen bond, occurs in various forms: hydrogen cyanide (volatile liquid that forms a gas at high temperatures) and sodium and potassium cyanide (salts). Cyanogen chloride (strong-smelling colorless liquified gas) can generate cyanide. Cyanide is used in some pesticides and fumigants (farm work, pest-control), in industrial processes (iron/steel), electroplating (jewelers), in wastewater treatment, in photo developing, in manufacturing (dyes, drugs), and in mining. Exposure per inhalation poses the greatest risk but cyanide can be absorbed through ingestion or contact with skin and eyes:

- **Low concentrations:** The body converts cyanide to thiocyanate and excretes in the urine. Patients may exhibit weakness, nausea, vomiting, eye irritation.
- **High concentrations**: The body can no longer compensate and hemoglobin is unable to uptake oxygen and tissue metabolism is inhibited, resulting in damage to the heart, lungs, and central nervous system. Patients may rapidly lose consciousness and die.

Reversal agents include inhaled amyl nitrite and IV sodium nitrite to form methemoglobin to trap cyanide and sodium thiosulfate to increase rate of conversion to thiocyanate. Skin should be flushed with water if contaminated and eyes flushed. If swallowed, the patient should drink large quantities of water and have vomiting induced.

HYDROGEN SULFIDE

Hydrogen sulfide, a colorless flammable gas with a strong "rotten egg" odor, occurs in petroleum, natural gas, hot springs, and the breakdown of sewage. Olfactory fatigue may occur rapidly, so the smell may be undetected. Heavier than air, hydrogen sulfide tends to collect in poorly-ventilated low-lying areas, such as basements, sewer lines, and manholes. Exposure is per inhalation and contact (eyes) and may affect the respiratory and central nervous systems:

- **Low concentrations**: Irritation to eyes (conjunctivitis, photophobia, tearing), nose, and respiratory system, resulting in burning, coughing, and dyspnea.
- **Moderate concentrations**: More severe irritation, dyspnea, pulmonary edema (with prolonged exposure at 250 ppm), headaches, dizziness, unstable gait, nausea and vomiting.
- **High concentrations**: Shock, seizures, respiratory distress, coma, and death. Effects may result from even one breath at high concentrations.

Preventive measures include monitoring, ventilating, and using appropriate protective gear, including impervious clothing, gloves, face shields (at least 8-inch) and approved respirators. Emergency treatment includes flushing eyes, flushing skin, oxygen, and CPR as necessary. Patients typically require high flow oxygen, and some may need positive pressure ventilation, IV fluids, vasopressors, correction of abnormal blood gas levels, induced methemoglobinemia, and/or hyperbaric oxygen therapy.

Chlorine

Chlorine (Cl) is a chemical element (amber liquid or green-yellow gas with strong odor) used in bleaches and disinfectants and in the chemical industry as a reagent, including manufacturing of polyvinyl chloride and other plastics. Chlorine by itself is highly poisonous, and the gas is denser than air, so it tends to accumulate near the ground level. Exposure is through contact with skin or eyes, or through inhalation. Symptoms include:

- **Short-term**: Liquid chlorine may cause burns and eye/skin irritation (blisters, inflammation, burning, tearing), especially at high concentrations. Inhaled chlorine may cause coughing, choking, chest pain, dyspnea, upper airway swelling, and pneumonia. High concentrations may result in death.
- **Long-term:** Tooth corrosion and skin irritation (acne), chest pain, cough, hemoptysis.

Preventive measures include appropriate engineering controls and the use of approved respirators, impervious clothing, glove, face shields (at least 8-inch), and safety goggles. Emergency treatment for contact with liquid chlorine includes immediate washing/showering. Eyes should be flushed with large amounts of water. If chlorine penetrates clothing, the clothing must be removed and skin flushed. If exposed to inhaled gas, oxygen should be administered and CPR provided if indicated. Treatment may include ventilation, nebulized sodium bicarbonate, and corticosteroids.

Toluene Diisocyanate

Toluene diisocyanates (TDI), which contain two isocyanate groups and are the most commonly used isocyanates, are chemicals used in manufacturing of polyurethanes, foams (rigid and flexible), varnishes, elastomers, adhesives, coatings, and sealants. TDIs are used in manufacturing of furniture, carpets, and bedding. Exposure is per ingestion, inhalation, or contact:

- **Short-term:** Contact result in severe skin irritation (erythema, blistering, edema) and eye irritation, which can cause permanent damage. Ingestion may result in nausea, vomiting, and abdominal pain. Inhalation may result in cough, chest pain, tightness in chest, headache, pulmonary edema, bronchospasm, insomnia. Some may develop an acute asthmatic reaction with reexposure.
- **Chronic**: Nocturnal coughing, dyspnea, and skin sensitization.

Preventive measures include engineering controls, chemical protective clothing, gloves, face shields (at least 8-inch), approved respirator, and safety goggles. Contaminated clothing should be removed, bagged and discarded or properly decontaminated (soaked in solution of 10% ammonia) and laundered. Emergency treatment includes showering and washing with soap and water. For eye exposure, eyes should be flushed for 15 minutes. For inhalation, treatment includes oxygen, bronchodilators, and corticosteroids. For ingestion, water is given to dilute along with activated charcoal (but no emesis). Gastric lavage is used only for large ingested quantities.

Ethylene Oxide

Ethylene oxide, a highly flammable gas with a sweet ether-like odor at room temperature and a liquid at below 51 °F, is used to manufacture antifreeze and as a chemical sterilant for foods and medical equipment. Ethylene oxide is heavier than air and accumulates in low-lying areas. Exposure is per inhalation of gas or contact with solution. Symptoms include:

- **Acute**: Irritation of skin, eyes, upper respiratory tract and inflammation of the trachea and bronchi, bronchial narrowing, partial lung collapse, pulmonary edema (may occur up to 72 hours after exposure), nausea, and vomiting. High concentrations may cause CNS depression with seizures, loss of consciousness, and coma (onset of neurological system may occur after 6 hours). Respiratory paralysis, cyanosis, renal damage, and peripheral nerve damage may occur.
- **Chronic**: Delayed peripheral nerve damage, impaired cognition, kidney and liver damage. Skin allergies and sensitization. Workers exposed to ethylene oxide may have increased risk of leukemia, cataracts, and birth defects in children.

Preventive measures include chemical protective clothing, approved respirators (positive-pressure, self-contained breathing apparatus), and gloves. Emergency treatment includes removing contaminated clothing and discarding, showering and washing with soap and water. Eyes should be flushed for 15 minutes. No antidote is available, so treatment is primarily supportive.

Organophosphates

Organophosphates are manufactured chemicals that are used to control insects and mammals in commercial agriculture and home gardening. They are most commonly used (comprising about one-half of killing agents) in insecticides, such as malathion, diazinon, parathion, ethion, dichlorvos, and chlorpyrifos. Organophosphates are also in nerve agents, and they have similar effects in pesticides, inhibiting acetylcholinesterase. Organophosphates can be inhaled, ingested, or absorbed through the skin. Symptoms of exposure include nausea, vomiting, diarrhea, abdominal cramping, miosis, tearing, sweating, salivating, bronchorrhea, wheezing, dyspnea, seizures, and severe muscle weakness. Patients may exhibit tachycardia and then bradycardia, and muscle weakness may lead to respiratory arrest and death. Nasogastric lavage and activated charcoal may be used for ingestion. Skin contamination should be treated by repeated washing with soap and water and dilute hypochlorite solution (1:10). Antidotes include atropine (which does not affect muscle weakness) and pralidoxime (which does), but treatment should be initiated as soon as possible after exposure to reverse damage.

Routes of Exposure to Workplace Chemicals

In the workplace, there are typically three different ways that a chemical can enter the body (called **routes of exposure**). They are inhalation (breathing), dermal (skin) absorption, and oral ingestion (swallowing).

Inhalation

Of the three, **inhalation** is the most common. Gases, mists, vapors, and airborne particles can all be inhaled, causing damage to the respiratory tract ranging from irritation to the lungs and throat, to more serious damage such as acute pneumonitis and pulmonary edema. When an inhaled chemical passes from the lungs to the bloodstream, there is the potential for systemic poisoning. Depending on the solubility of the inhaled chemical, the effects can be felt immediately (as in the highly soluble gases hydrogen fluoride, ammonia, and sulfuric acid), or several hours later (for less soluble gases such as nitrogen dioxide and phosgene).

Nose vs. Mouth Breathing

The switch from nose breathing to mouth breathing changes the anatomy of the **respiratory tract** in a subtle but important way. Because the nasal hairs of the nasopharynx remove some of the larger particles that are inhaled, they can be considered the body's natural air filters. Although it is limited in the amount that is actually filtered, there is a decrease in the number of particles that reach the lungs. When one breathes by mouth, the nasopharynx is bypassed, allowing more particles directly into the lungs for absorption. Chemicals that are inhaled exert their toxicity when they are absorbed by the tissue of the lungs and then distributed to the rest of the body. Thus, because more particles are delivered to the lungs with mouth breathing, the toxicity of the chemical increases.

Dermal Absorption

In **dermal absorption**, chemicals are absorbed through the skin. The skin is the body's first line of defense from exposure to harmful substances, and so it is made up of many layers of cells. For this reason, dermal absorption of a chemical is not considered a major route of exposure. The ability of a chemical to get through the layers of skin and be absorbed into the body depends on factors such as the kind of chemical, length of time of the exposure, and the presence of cuts or other open wounds on the skin.

Oral Ingestion

Of all possible routs of exposure, **oral ingestion** of a chemical is the least likely to occur in the workplace. If it does happen, it is either through eating or drinking contaminated food or water, or a chemical is swallowed after it has entered the mouth due to inhalation. Certain behaviors or activities, such as mouth breathing, chewing gum or tobacco, or placing fingers or tools in the mouth, increase a person's risk of exposure to chemicals through oral ingestion. If a chemical is ingested, the acids in the stomach can help to reduce its toxicity.

Injection

Injection is one of four major routes of exposure to chemical hazards (inhalation, contact, ingestion, injection). Injection most commonly occurs in treatment when toxic medications, such as chemotherapeutic agents, are administered and in needlestick injuries. If a healthcare provider experiences a needlestick injury, the initial response should be to wash the wound with soap and water. As soon as possible, the incident must be reported to a supervisor and steps taken according to established protocol. This may include testing and/or prophylaxis, depending on the patient's health history. In some cases, the patient may also be tested for communicable diseases, such as HIV, in order to determine the risk to the injured party. PEP (post-exposure prophylaxis) is available for exposure to HIV (human immunodeficiency virus) and HBV (hepatitis B virus). However, no PEP is available for HCV (hepatitis C virus) although the CDC does provide a plan for management. PEP should be initiated within 72 hours of exposure. All testing and treatments associated with the needlestick injury must be provided free of cost.

OSHA Standard's (HCS 2012) Classification of Specific Organ Toxicity

OSHA through the Hazard Communication Standard (HCS) utilizes the **specific target organ toxicity (STOT) classification** to indicate how chemicals affect different organ systems:

- **Single exposure (STOT-SE):** Category 1 substances may produce significant toxicity; Category 2 substances may be harmful to human health. Category 1 and 2 indications may include functional changes; adverse change in clinical biochemistry, hematology, or urinalysis; organ damage; necrosis; granuloma formation; and morphological changes. Category 3 may have transient target organ effects. Category 3 indications may include cough, edema, pruritis, pain, inflammation, central nervous system depression.

- **Repeated/Prolonged exposure (STOT-RE)**: Category 1 substances produce significant toxicity; Category 2 substances may be harmful to human health. Most chemicals with organ toxicity are in Category 1 with indications similar to those of single exposure except that repeated or prolonged exposure is required.

Effects of Chemical Agents on Pregnancy

Chemical exposure can adversely affect the sperm, egg, or fetus. Damage to any of these can result in infertility, birth defects, spontaneous abortion, and heritable genetic defects. The gravity of the effect depends greatly on the timing of the exposure. There are many chemicals that have a known/suspected effect on pregnancy. The suspected **effects on pregnancy** of each of the following chemical agents are as follows:

- **Heavy Metals**: Neurological and behavioral deficits in infants.
- **Organic solvents**: Spontaneous abortion, moderate increase in risk of birth defects, fetal solvent syndrome.
- **Antineoplastic Agents**: Spontaneous abortion.
- **Antivirals**: Spontaneous abortion, sperm effects in males, teratogenesis in females.
- **Estrogenic/Antiestrogenic Compounds**: Spontaneous abortion, sperm effects in males, teratogenesis in females.
- **Immunosuppressive Agents**: Spontaneous abortion, sperm effects in males, teratogenesis in females.
- **Carcinogens and Mutagens**: Sperm effects in males, teratogenesis and cancer in the offspring of exposed females.
- **Waste Anesthetic Gases**: Spontaneous abortion.
- **Sterilants and Disinfectants**: Spontaneous abortion.
- **Polychlorinated Biphenyls (PCBs)**: Congenital PCB syndrome, mild neonatal growth, behavioral deficits.
- **Pesticides**: Both male and female reproductive effects.

Perinatal Toxicology

Perinatal toxicology is the study of the toxic response to chemical agents when the time of exposure is between conception and one month after birth. Because this timeframe exhibits many different stages of development, the gravity of a toxic response varies based on the timing of the exposure. Thus, in order to fully understand the effects of toxic chemicals on the reproductive system, it is necessary to understand the effects of chemical exposure relative to the stage of gestational development. Some potential **toxic responses bases on gestation** are as follows:

- **Implantation (6-7 days)**: embryonic death.
- **Organogenesis (7days-2 months)**: birth defects.
- **Embryonic Period (0-3 months)**: birth defects.
- **Fetal Period (3-9 months):** developmental and behavioral deficits, endocrine and immune dysfunction, cancer.
- **Neonatal Period (after birth)**: functional deficits.

Teratogenesis

Teratogenesis is the development of birth defects while in the womb (in utero) as a result of exposure to a toxic substance. Teratogens cause defects in what would otherwise be healthy tissue. While the exact mechanisms of teratogenesis are not known, it is hypothesized that some possible causes include the inhibition of DNA and RNA, changes in the structural formation of nucleic acids, or the inhibition of certain enzymes. Dose is an important factor in teratogenesis. If the exposure dose is high, the result is spontaneous abortion/embryonic death. If the dose is low, there is often no observable affect to the fetus. Thus, it is a relatively exact dose that can cause teratogenesis, and this depends on the overall toxicity of the chemical.

Chemicals That Can Cause Adverse Reproductive Outcomes

Many chemicals are known to cause **adverse reproductive outcomes**. The following are some of those **outcomes** and the **chemicals** that can cause each:

- **Infertility**: anesthetic agents, cadmium, chloroprene, ethylene dibromide, lead, manganese
- **Male fecundity**: boron, cadmium, carbon disulfide, chloroprene, ethylene dibromide, lead, manganese
- Female fecundity: mercury
- **Menstrual disorders**: aniline, benzene, carbon disulfide, chloroprene, formaldehyde, lead, toluene
- **Prematurity/low birth weight**: cadmium, CO, formaldehyde, mercury, toluene, vinyl chloride
- **Spontaneous abortion/stillbirth**: anesthetic agents, antineoplastics, arsenic, carbon disulfide, chloroprene, ethylene oxide, lead, vinyl chloride
- **Birth defects**: antineoplastics, benzene, lead
- **Contaminated breast milk**: benzene, cadmium, DDT, dieldrin, lead, mercury

Chemicals Suspected to Affect Male Reproductive Function

The **chemicals** that have suspected **effects on male reproductive function** are as follows:

- **Decreased libido/hormonal alterations**: lead, mercury, manganese, carbon disulfide, estrogen agonists.
- **Sperm toxicity**: lead, DBCP, carbaryl, toluene diamine, dinitrotoluene, ethylene dibromide, styrene, acetone, ethylene glycol monoethyl ether, welding, perchloroethylene, mercury, heat military radar, Kepone, bromine, radiation, carbon disulfide, 2,4-dichlorophenoxy.
- Spontaneous abortion in partner: solvents, lead, mercury.
- **Altered sex ratio in offspring**: dibromochloropropane (DBCP).
- **Congenital malformations in offspring**: pesticides, chlorophenates, solvents.
- **Neurobehavioral disorders in offspring**: alcohols, cyclophosphamide, ethylene bromide, lead, opiates.
- **Childhood cancer in offspring**: solvents, paints, pesticides, petroleum products.

Preventing Reproductive Disorders Caused by Workplace Exposures

The **prevention of reproductive disorders** due to exposures to toxic chemicals is an important aspect of an environmental health and safety program. There are several ways to reduce the risk of exposure to chemicals that have the potential to have negative reproductive effects. Regular worksite inspections are a must. If a hazardous situation is identified, engineering and administrative controls should be employed to remediate the problem. To understand the reproductive health of the workforce, a reproductive health survey should be included in a standard occupational health history. And, as always, education of the workforce should be a key part of an occupational health and safety program. Workers need to fully understand the reproductive risks associated with the chemicals in the workplace. Safety Data Sheets (SDS) can help with this understanding. Thus, both management and workers need to know where SDS are located, as well as the information they contain.

Latex Allergy

Latex sensitivity is increasing in frequency, especially among those who are exposed to latex regularly through work, such as rubber industry workers, or have repeated contact with the healthcare system. Contact through direct touching can result in cutaneous, mucosal, or percutaneous exposure. Parenteral exposure may be related to IVs with latex ports or injections into system with syringes containing dry latex. Latex Foley catheters are another common source of this allergic response in the health care environment. Inhalation can result from inhaling protein particles from someone in the room using powdered latex gloves. Latex sensitivity may manifest as 3 different types of reactions:

- **Irritant** (non-immune): Erythematous irritation from contact. Treatment includes antihistamines.
- **Contact dermatitis** (type 4): Dry erythema beyond area of contact with pruritis, weeping, and blistering and results from chemicals (thiurams and thiazoles) used in production of latex. Treatment includes antihistamines and topical hydrocortisone.
- **IgE** (type I) (immune reaction): Response to proteins in latex with urticaria, rhinitis, angioedema, asthma, laryngeal edema, anaphylactic shock, and death. Treatment includes:
    - Establish patent airway and intubate if necessary for ventilation, high flow oxygen (100%).
    - Administer epinephrine. Albuterol per nebulizer for bronchospasm.
    - Intravenous fluids to provide bolus of fluids for hypotension.
    - Diphenhydramine if shock persists. Methylprednisolone if no response to other drugs.

Ranking System for Acute Chemical Toxicity

The following is the ranking system for **acute chemical toxicity**, given in the following format: Class - Lethal Dose for an adult - Example

1. **Practically Nontoxic** - >15g/kg (more than one quart) - Sugar
2. **Slightly Toxic** - 5-15g/kg (between one pint and one quart) - Salt
3. **Moderately Toxic** - 0.5-5g/kg (between one ounce and one pint) - 2,4-D (herbicide)
4. **Very Toxic** - 50-500mg/kg (between one teaspoonful and one ounce) - Arsenic Acid
5. **Extremely Toxic** - 5-50mg/kg (between 7 drops and one teaspoonful) - Nicotine
6. **Supertoxic** - <5mg/kg (<7 drops) - Botulism Toxin

Influences on Chemical Toxicity

Age

Aside from the type of chemical, dose, and route of exposure, there are other factors that influence the level of toxicity of a chemical. **Age** is one of these factors. Infants and children are at a higher risk of experiencing a toxic effect than adults due to the immaturity and resulting inability of their organs to adequately filter out toxic substances. Furthermore, because they are growing and going through a great deal of cell division, there is a greater chance that a chemical will have a carcinogenic effect. The extremely young are not the only ones at a higher risk of realizing the toxic effects of chemicals. Due to the deterioration of filtering organs and an overall reduction in healing time, older workers are also at risk to experience the harmful effects of a chemical exposure.

Gender

Chemical exposure can adversely affect the sperm, egg, or fetus. Damage to any of these can result in infertility, birth defects, spontaneous abortion, and heritable genetic defects. The gravity of the effect depends greatly on the timing of the exposure. For example, during times of rapid cell division and differentiation, the fetus is much more susceptible to the negative effects of chemical exposure.

NUTRITION

The process of breaking down and eliminating toxins from the body is called biotransformation. In order for this process to proceed in a timely fashion (thus limiting the length of exposure and potential damage a chemical can cause), certain key enzymes are necessary. The existence of these enzymes (which are proteins) in the body is directly linked to diet. A good, healthful diet is what supplies the substances necessary for the biotransformation process. Without the biotransformation process, toxins would build up in the body, resulting in illness or death.

HEALTH STATUS

Depending on an individual's health, a toxic chemical can have a greater or lesser effect on them. For example, if a person's health is compromised in ways such as liver, lung, or immunologic disease, exposure to a toxic chemical would have a more severe effect than in a healthy individual. Unhealthy lifestyle habits, such as drinking, smoking, or being overweight, can increase the possibility of a person developing a disease or illness when exposed to toxic chemicals.

INDIVIDUAL SUSCEPTIBILITY

Not everyone responds to chemicals in the same way. A chemical that has a high level of toxicity for one person may not be the same for another. Individual susceptibility is a phenomenon in which the immune system mounts a response even if the exposure levels are low. This is called hypersensitivity. In some instances, an individual can have a reaction to a chemical at an exposure level that is considered "safe." For this reason, everyone must be aware of the chemicals being used in the workplace and the signs of toxic exposure.

WORKER HISTORY

In the case of repeat exposures, the potential for realizing the negative effects of a chemical often increase with repeat successive exposures. It is also possible that chemical exposure and any associated negative effects can have a long latency period, such that illness or disease is not evident for months or years. Thus, a substance may appear to be nontoxic, when in fact the opposite is true. This was the case with asbestos in the workplace. Finally, exposure to multiple different chemicals can have a greater effect on a worker than exposure to any of the chemicals individually. This can be the case whether the exposures were at the same time or at different times throughout the individual's work history.

Biologic Hazards

Biological Hazards in the Workplace

Biological hazards are biological substances/entities that pose a health risk in the workplace. Biological hazards can include pathogens (bacteria, fungi, viruses, parasites), animals, insects, sewage, plants, birds, feces/droppings, human beings as well as medical wastes. The types of biological hazards workers are exposed to varies according to the field of work. Healthcare providers, for example, are at increased risk primarily from medical wastes, pathogens, human beings, and needlestick injuries. Farmworkers are primarily at risk from insects, pathogens, birds, plants, and animals. Jobs that have increased risk also include cleaning services, garbage disposal, fishery work, veterinary services, manufacturing jobs (involving plant/animal raw materials), restaurant work, and jobs in enclosed facilities with central air conditioning. Each job should be assessed for potential biological hazards and steps taken to prevent risk through engineering controls (safety equipment, disinfecting, pesticide control, disposal protocols) and administrative controls (immunizations, sick leave, training). Various types of masks and respirators (N95, powered air purifying respirator, air-supply respirators) and protective clothing (coveralls, gowns, face shields, safety goggles, and gloves) may be utilized to prevent exposure.

Biologic Hazards

Tuberculosis

Tuberculosis (TB) is caused by *Mycobacterium tuberculosis* and there is an increase in resistant strains. TB is a particular danger to those who are immunocompromised, with 8-10% of those with HIV developing TB. Healthcare workers are also at risk. Patients with TB may develop weight loss, general debility, night sweats, and fever. With pulmonary involvement, a progressive cough resulting in dyspnea and bloody sputum is common. Diagnosis is per skin and sputum testing and x-ray. Transmission is from airborne particles, so anyone in contact to someone with active TB is at risk of inhaling particles. Precautions:

- Prompt diagnosis and anti-tuberculosis drugs.
- Airborne infection isolation (in a negative-pressure isolation room if available).
- Skin testing/x-rays of contacts.
- Preventive Isoniazid therapy for those with latent infection or newly converted to positive on TB testing.

Commonly used first-line drugs include isoniazid (INH) and rifampin. For latent TB Isoniazid (INH) for 9 months is the treatment of choice. Second-line drugs include amikacin, kanamycin, or capreomycin. Since the 1980s there has been increased need to use second-line drugs because of resistance. Causes for increased resistance:

- Failure to complete a course of treatment.
- Mismanaged treatment, including incorrect medication, dosage, or duration of therapy.

Tetanus

Tetanus is a life-threatening non-communicable bacterial infection caused by a spore found in soil, dust, and animal feces. Those at increased risk include farm workers, construction workers, campers, gardeners, and firefighters. The bacteria produce an endotoxin affecting the central nervous system. Transmission is through puncture wounds/breaks in the skin or through the umbilical cord after birth. Incubation period is 2 days to months (usually 2 weeks). Symptoms include neck and jaw stiffness, facial spasms, difficulty chewing and swallowing, headache, sensitivity to noise, painful muscle contractions at site of infection, opisthotonos (rigid hyperextension) positioning, and airway obstruction. Infants may be unable to suck. Complications include laryngospasm, respiratory distress, and death (30%). Preventive measures include tetanus immunizations and boosters every 10 years. Post-exposure if no immunization requires tetanus immune globulin and tetanus toxoid. Emergency care includes standard precautions, managing airway/ventilation/intubation and providing supplemental oxygen as needed, IV access line, and protection from injury.

Food and Waterborne Pathogens

Organism	***Vibrio parahaemolyticus***	***Vibrio cholerae***	***Campylobacter jejuni***	***Shigella sp.***
Onset	2 to 48 hours	24 to 72 hours	2 to 5 days	24 to 48 hours
Duration	2 to 5 days	Death may occur ≤18 hours without treatment.	2 to 10 days. Relapse may occur.	5 to 7 days
Source/ Exposure risk	Undercooked/raw Seafood.	Contaminated water, seafood, street food.	Undercooked/raw poultry, contaminated water, unpasteurized milk. Transmitted from pets to children.	Fecal-contaminated water or foods.
Signs and symptoms	Watery diarrhea, abdominal cramping, nausea, and vomiting. Onset is abrupt.	Severe copious liquid diarrhea with dehydration. Onset is abrupt.	Fever, abdominal cramping and bloody diarrhea. Associated with Guillain-Barre syndrome & Reiter's syndrome.	Bloody, purulent diarrhea, cramps, and lethargy. Onset is abrupt.
Treatment	Supportive	IV/oral fluid and electrolytes. Supportive care. Tetracyclines shorten duration	Supportive care. Erythromycin shortens duration.	Supportive care. Fluoroquinolones.

Escherichia Coli

Escherichia coli is part of the normal flora of the intestines and serves to inhibit other bacteria, but 5 serotypes can cause intestinal disease and severe diarrhea if ingested. Some types are more common in developing countries and may occur in people who are traveling in areas where feces have contaminated food supplies and water. Severe outbreaks of *E. coli* infection have occurred in the United States with a toxic strain, 0157:H7, which produces a toxin that can cause damage to the intestinal lining, including blood vessels, resulting in hemorrhage and watery diarrhea that becomes bloody, especially in children and the elderly. This hemorrhagic colitis usually clears with supportive treatment after 10 days. However, about 15% of children develop sepsis and hemolytic uremic syndrome with kidney failure, hemolytic anemia, and thrombocytopenia. Death rates are 3-5%, but residual renal and neurological damage may result. Treatment is supportive with intravenous therapy, blood transfusions, and kidney dialysis. Antibiotics and antidiarrheals are contraindicated as they may worsen *E. coli* infections.

Giardia Lamblia

Giardia lamblia is a protozoan that infects water supplies and spreads to adults and children through the fecal-oral route. It is the most common cause on non-bacterial diarrhea in the United States, causing about 20,000 cases of infection each year in all ages. Children often become infected swallowing recreational waters (pools, lakes) or putting contaminated items into the mouth. *Giardia* lives and multiplies within the small intestine where cysts develop. Symptoms occur 7-14 days after ingestion of 1 or more cysts and include: Diarrhea with greasy floating stools (rarely bloody), stomach cramps, nausea, and flatulence, lasting 2-6 weeks. Chronic infection may develop. *Diagnosis* is based on 3 stool specimens, ELISA, or PCR for DNA. Treatment includes:

- Metronidazole (Flagyl®) 250 mg 3 times daily for 5 days (drug of choice.
  - Pediatric dose: 15mg/kg/day in 3 doses for 5 days
- Nitazoxanide 500 mg twice daily for 3 days.
  - Pediatric dose: 1-3 years 100 mg every 12 hours for 3 days; 4-11 years 200 mg every 12 hours for 3 days.

Salmonella

Salmonella causes up to 4 million infections in the United States, resulting in 500 deaths, primarily of young children. *Salmonella* is spread by the fecal-oral route through ingestion of contaminated food or water, including all meats, milk, eggs, and vegetables, so food workers are at increased risk. Raw or undercooked meat, unpasteurized milk, and unwashed produce are high-risk. *Salmonella* may be found in the feces of pets, particularly reptiles such as snakes and turtles. Small children should not have reptiles as pets. Symptoms appear 12-72 hours after infection and include bloody diarrhea with abdominal pain, fever, and vomiting. Most cases resolve within 7-10 days, but in some cases, life-threatening sepsis may occur, requiring treatment with antibiotics. Amoxicillin 40 g/kg/day in 3 doses for 7-10 days is the antibiotic of choice. Antibiotic prophylaxis is usually contraindicated except in children <1 year that are at risk for bacteremia or those who are immunocompromised.

Bloodborne Pathogens

HIV

HIV (human immunodeficiency virus) is the retrovirus that causes AIDS (acquired immune deficiency syndrome). Diagnosis is determined by the CD4+ T-cell count with AIDS currently diagnosed with a CD4+ count of <200 cells per mm^3 and an AIDS defining condition, such as opportunistic infections (cytomegalovirus, tuberculosis), wasting syndrome, neoplasms (Kaposi's sarcoma), or AIDS dementia complex. HIV is transmitted in bodily fluids (blood, semen, vaginal secretions, breast milk) that contain free virions and infected CD4+ T-cells. About 1.2 million people in the United States have HIV infection but 13% are unaware of infection. HIV immunocompromised patients are susceptible to contracting infectious diseases. HIV-related pneumonia is most often caused by *Pneumocystis jiroveci,* but fungal pneumonias are also prevalent among patients with HIV. Tuberculosis is a particular danger to those who are immunocompromised, with 8-10% of those with HIV developing TB. Risk factors include unprotected sex, especially males having sex with other males, and needle sharing. Emergency care: supportive care, manage airway, support ventilation, IV access if necessary. Droplet precautions for cough. Treatment: antiretroviral agents (NRTIs, NNRTIs, protease inhibitors, fusion inhibitors, integrase strand transfer inhibitor, and multiclass combination products).

Hepatitis B

Hepatitis B (HBV), the most common blood-borne hepatitis, is transmitted in body fluids (blood, semen, and vaginal fluids) and through needle sharing and is very infectious, resulting in both acute and chronic infections. Most recover within 6 months but up to 10% develop chronic disease, which can lead to liver failure and or liver cancer, and become carriers. HBV vaccination, the best preventive, is recommended for all newborns as well as all those<18 and those in high-risk groups >18 (drug users, men having sex with men, those with multiple sex partners, partners of those with HBV, healthcare workers, and older adults with end-stage renal disease, chronic liver disease, or HIV/AIDS and in correctional or drug-abuse treatment facilities). Incidence is highest among drug-using adults 30 to 39 years. Preventive treatment also includes immunoglobulin injection within 12 hours of exposure. Treatment for infection includes antiviral medications to slow progression, interferon alfa-2b injections (usually reserved for young adults), and liver transplant if liver failure occurs. There is no curative treatment. Healthcare providers should wear PPE and care for patients in dedicated isolation rooms with dedicated equipment (including instruments and supplies) and should not also care for patients who are susceptible (HBSag/HBSAB negative).

Animal Hazards

Animal hazards may vary widely and can include:

- Animal attacks: Scratches, bites, fractures, mauling, and infections.
- Enclosure injuries: Cuts, infections.
- Wastes/Feces/Droppings: Infections, eye, skin, and upper respiratory irritation.
- Handling: Musculoskeletal injuries, strains, sprains.
- Zoonoses: Infections (Q fever, ringworm, rabies, salmonella, psittacosis).
- Allergic response: Rhinitis, pruritis, asthma.
- Eye injuries: Dust, foreign bodies, airborne contaminants.
- Heat/Cold stress: Protective clothing/Environment too hot or too cold.
- Excess noise: Barking or other loud noises.

Work environments that increase risk include veterinary services, animal shelters, agricultural/farm work, and research facilities (involving animals). Preventive measures include frequent hand hygiene and use of personal protective clothing and equipment, safety glasses, protective footwear, hearing protection, ergonomics training, heat/cold precautions, and adequate hydration. Employers should provide PPE, training, and hand-washing/sanitation equipment. Those working directly with animals that may develop rabies (cats, dogs, ferrets) should have preexposure rabies vaccinations. Any worker with bites or other injuries should seek prompt medical evaluation and treatment to prevent further complications.

BIOTERRORISM

Bioterrorism is the use of biological agents (viruses, bacteria, fungi) to attack and cause illness, death, or contamination in people, air supplies, water supplies, animals, and/or crops. There are similar steps to take regardless of the pathogen. There are a number of different infections that could be part of a bioterrorism attack, such as smallpox, *Bacillus anthracis* (anthrax), *Clostridium botulinum*, *Francisella tularensis* (tularemia) and *Yersinia pestis* (pneumonic plague). Procedure for suspected bioterrorism:

- Be on the alert for possible bioterrorism-related infections, based on clusters of patients or symptoms.
- Use personal protection equipment, including respirators when indicated.
- Complete thorough assessment of patient, including medical history, physical examination, immunization record, and travel history.
- Provide a probable diagnosis based on symptoms and lab findings, including cultures.
- Provide treatment, including prophylaxis while waiting for laboratory findings.
- Use transmission precautions as well as isolation for suspected biologic agents.
- Notify local, state, and federal authorities as per established protocol.
- Conduct surveillance and epidemiological studies to identify at risk populations.
- Develop plans to accommodate large numbers of patients: Restricting elective admissions, transferring patients, and reutilizing existing facilities.

TRAVEL MEDICINE

Travel medicine focuses on the preventive care for people who are traveling and putting themselves at risk of disease and for the people and area the travelers are visiting. Travel medicine includes:

- Conducting risk assessments to determine what diseases or conditions may be impacted by travel or encountered, including risks of communicable diseases (coronavirus infection, dengue, malaria, hepatitis, tuberculosis, leishmaniasis).
- Discussing risks associated with flying, including transmission of infectious diseases among passengers sitting in close proximity to each other (especially a concern for immunocompromised patients).
- Assessing the need for vaccinations required or recommended for different destinations, such as the yellow fever vaccination if traveling to areas of Africa and South America, and rabies pre- and post-exposure vaccinations (India, Southeast Asia).
- Prescribing preventive medications or self-treatment regimens for those traveling to areas where disease is endemic, such as traveler's diarrhea (*E. coli*).
- Assessing the risks associated with travel to areas with high levels of air and/or water pollution. Air pollution may seriously impact heart and lung function for those with cardiopulmonary disease.

Physical Hazards/Ergonomics

Occupational Noise

According to **OSHA's Noise Standard** (29 CFR 1910.95) a noise abatement program must be in place if workers are exposed to time-weighted average noise levels of 85 decibels (dBA) during an 8-hour period of work. The exposure limit is 90 dBA/8 hr, and for every 5 dBA above 90, the time of exposure must be reduced by half. Thus for 95 dBA, exposure is limited to 4 hours. Levels above 55 dBA impact the ability to hear and understand spoken communication. High levels of noise and extended durations of exposure may result in hearing loss, tinnitus, anxiety, fatigue, stress, and GI problems and is linked to high cholesterol and hypertension. Employers should monitor noise levels with a sound meter and identify any equipment or processes that have increased levels of noise. Methods of reducing noise include:

- Providing personal protection equipment, such as earplugs and noise-cancelling earphones.
- Using equipment that generates lower dBA.
- Utilizing engineering controls: Sound barriers, sound dampeners, acoustical wall/ceiling tiles.
- Utilizing administrative controls: Training, job rotation.
- Moving noise-generating equipment, such as compressors, out of the immediate work area.

Occupational Vibration

Some equipment, such as chainsaws. grinders, air-powered wrenches, dental tools, and stone-chipping tools, produce both noise and **vibration**, and when the two are combined, the risk of hearing loss increases. However, vibration alone also has negative effects on the musculoskeletal system, and can result in hand-arm vibration syndrome (HAVS) and Raynaud's phenomenon of occupational origin, which can cause impaired circulation (vibration white finger), damage to sensory nerves, and damage to bones, joints, and muscles, and whole-body vibration (WBV). WBV is often associated with low back pain and other injuries. Vibration decreases circulation, resulting in vascular and nerve damage. Manuals for tools should provide information about the amplitude of vibration although this information relates to new tools, and older tools may cause more vibration. (OSHA has not yet established acceptable vibration limits.) In the early stages of vibration syndromes, patients may experience persistent numbness and tingling, increasing to blanching and pain. Preventive measures include anti-vibration equipment, engineering controls to limit use, training and education, 10-minute breaks each hour, avoiding chill and wearing appropriate clothing to maintain body temperature, and grasping vibrating tools lightly.

Sources of Occupational Radiation

Ionizing Radiation

Atoms contain a nucleus with protons and neutrons, surrounded by electrons. The number of protons determines the element; and the number of neutrons, the isotopes. Unstable isotopes decay (give off radiation) to stabilize, rendering them radioactive. If the radiation is strong enough to ionize (remove negatively-charged electrons it encounters), it is **ionizing radiation**. Ionizing radiation may occur in uranium and radium, or in accelerators and reactors. Some equipment, including x-ray machines, produce ionizing radiation. There are different types of ionizing radiation: particulate radiation (alpha, beta, positrons, and neutrons) and electromagnetic radiation (gamma rays, x-rays). The Nuclear Regulatory Commission and OSHA regulate ionizing radiation. OSHA standards for ionizing body can receive: 18.75 rem/quarter to hands/forearms and feet/ankles, 7.5 rem/quarter to all of skin, and 1.25 rem/quarter to whole body (head and trunk, blood-forming organs, eye lens, gonads). Occupations/Areas at risk include medicine (CT scans, x-rays, nuclear medicine, fluoroscopy), general industry, construction, shipyard employment, marine terminals, and longshoring. Preventive measures include restricting access, barriers, and PPE. Employers must ensure dose limits are not exceeded, must monitor for radiation hazards, provide personal monitoring dosimeters, provide safety/caution signage, and provide training and instruction regarding operating procedures.

Lasers

Lasers are strong beams of light used in surgical procedures and industrial processes. Lasers provide directional rather than diffuse (spreading) light. Use of lasers is regulated under OSHA's general industry standards (29 CFR 1910) and guidance provided by the American National Standards Institute. The FDA (21 CFR 1040) provides standards for lasers; and the National Fire Protection Association is the standard for fire protection as lasers pose a risk of fire. Injuries related to laser radiation are primarily thermal, resulting in burn injuries to the eyes or skin with the risk increasing as the intensity of the laser increases. When used for surgery, laser-retardant drapes should be used and wet dressings placed on the drapes about the surgical site. Flammable solutions, such as alcohol, should be avoided. Halon fire extinguishers should be available. To prevent injury, laser beams should be directed horizontally and not at eye level. Those exposed to lasers should use protective goggles. Work spaces may be protected by laser safety windows and barriers.

Infrared Light

Most **infrared radiation exposure** is from the sun, but thermal waves produced in industry and some devices also generate infrared radiation. Infrared light is not visible but is perceived as heat. Infrared light has a longer wavelength (700 nm-1 mm) than visible light, and a lower frequency (430 THz-300GHz). Industries that pose special risks include steel (heated metal) and glass blowing (molten glass) as well as outdoor work, such as gardening. Other common sources of infrared radiation include radiant heaters, welding equipment, furnaces, and electrical appliances. The skin and the eyes (photochemical injury) are especially susceptible to injury from infrared radiation, with damage increasing with wavelength. Prolonged exposure to infrared radiation may result in the development of cataracts. Preventive measures include eliminating or reducing infrared exposure, engineering controls (matte finishes to prevent reflection, curtains, filters, warning signs), PPE (protective clothing, safety glasses, face shields, gloves).

Microwaves

Microwave radiation is a form of high-frequency electromagnetic radiation that is generated from radios, cell phones, cooking, processing foods, heat sealers, welders, induction heaters, and communications and radar transmitters. Microwave is used for limited sterilization of compatible medical devices, such as dentures, urinary catheters (for self-catheterization), contact lenses, and dental instruments. Microwave diathermy is used to increase the temperature in subcutaneous tissue, muscles, and joints and should not be directed at areas where increased temperatures may be detrimental. Microwaves are absorbed in a manner similar to light. Microwave devices may leak radiation and cause fires. Exposure to microwaves can result in burns and tissue damage. The eyes and testes are especially vulnerable because of limited ability to dissipate heat. Exposure to high microwave levels may lead to cataracts. Preventive measures include the use of microwave radiation shields/protection devices (aluminum foil, metal foam, sheet metal), and maintaining appropriate distance from source.

NRC and Radiation Exposure Reduction

The U.S. Congress gave the **Nuclear Regulatory Commission** (NRC) authority to protect the population and environment from unnecessary exposure to radiation resulting from civilian use.

The NRC has regulations regarding nuclear power plants, research reactions, and medical, industrial, and academic licenses regarding the use and storage of radioactive materials. NRC sets dose limits and requires users to obtain licenses and to submit to inspections. The NRC shares regulatory authority with the EPA (air emission and water standards for radioisotopes) and the FDA (standards for nuclear medicine procedures). The NRC regulates source materials (uranium, thorium), special nuclear material, and byproducts (10 CFR, part 20):

- Dose limits for workers and public.
- Exposure limits for individual radionuclides.
- Monitoring and labeling of radioactive materials.
- Signage around radiation areas.
- Reporting procedures for theft/loss of radioactive materials.
- Penalties for noncompliance.

The NRC provides technical support to state regulatory programs as well as a database regarding regulatory information and enters agreements with state governors to authorize states to regulate some radioactive materials within the state, such as those used in medicine and industry. States are required to use the same standards as the NRC.

Green Job Hazards

Heat

Heat Stress

Increased temperature causes dehydration. Symptoms may include swelling of hands and feet, flushing, itching, sunburn, dizziness, muscle cramps, and hyperventilation. Temperature is normal.

Emergency treatment:

- Remove from heat and give fluids to rehydrate, oxygen with non-rebreather mask.

Heat Exhaustion

Dehydration results in sodium depletion. Symptoms may include flu-like symptoms, headache, dizziness, fainting, nausea, vomiting, weakness, muscle cramping, rapid pulse, diaphoresis, cold clammy skin. Temperature usually <106 °F (41 °C) and may be normal.

Emergency treatment:

- Remove from heat, evaporative cooling techniques ice packs to axilla, groin, neck, rehydrate (1/2 glass every 15 to 20 minutes). Oxygen with non-rebreather mask.

Heat Stroke

Two types of heat stroke may progress to multi-organ dysfunction syndrome with liver and kidney failure, and death:

- **Exertional** – Sudden onset after exertion, temperature varies because still sweating, diaphoresis, syncope, loss of consciousness.
- **Non-exertional** – Sudden onset after heat exposure, temperature usually >106 °F (41 °C) rectally or >103 °F (39.4 °C) orally, mild irritability, decorticate posturing, seizures, to coma, tachycardia.

Emergency treatment:

- Remove from heat, evaporative cooling and ice packs as above, airway/ventilation/oxygenation support as needed, IV access line and fluids, rapid transport.

Cold Stress

Workers involved in green jobs may be exposed to extremes of weather, resulting in **cold stress.** Risk factors include being wet/damp, wearing inadequate clothing, being exhausted, having predisposing health conditions (hypothyroidism, diabetes mellitus, hypertension) and being in poor physical condition. Cold stress:

- **Trench foot:** Occurs when feet are constantly wet, resulting in heat loss, erythema, tingling, pain, blisters, leg cramps, and numbness. Treatment includes drying and elevating feet.
- **Frostbite:** Tissue damage from freezing (especially nose, ears, and distal extremities). The affected part feels numb and aches or throbs, becoming hard and insensate as tissue freezes, resulting in circulatory impairment, necrosis of tissue, and gangrene. Treatment as for hypothermia.
- **Hypothermia:** Core body temperature <35 °C, resulting in uncontrollable shivering, pallor altered level of consciousness, slurred speech, tachycardia, bradypnea, coma, and death. Treatment:
    - **Stage I** (mild) hypothermia (CBT 32-35 °C): Dry, warm clothes, and passive external warming (warm drinks, warmed blankets, warm baths at 40 °C, and physical activity). **Stage II** (moderate) hypothermia (CBT 28-32 °C.) and **stage III** (severe) hypothermia (24-28 °C): Passive and active warming, such as warm intravenous fluids (38-42 °C), warm humidified oxygen or air inhalation, warming with extracorporeal circuit, and internal (bladder, peritoneal pleural, GI) lavage, as indicated.

Electrical Hazards

The Occupational Safety and Health Administration (OSHA) lists the **electrical hazards** that result in most electrical injuries:

- **Contact with power lines (overhead and buried):** May result in electrocution, burns, and falls. Workers/Others should stay at least 10 feet way from overhead powerlines, should contact power companies for locations of buried lines, de-energize and ground wires when working near them, and use non-conductive wood or fiberglass ladders.
- **Lack of ground-fault protection**: Without protection, a current can go through a worker's body.
- **Path to ground missing or discontinuous**: Moisture must be avoided at cord connectors, and cords must be inspected for insulation breaks.
- **Equipment not used in prescribed manner:** Tools should be used according to directions and should be double-insulated and visually inspected before use.
- **Improper use of extension and flexible cords**: Flexible cords must be connected so there is no tension at joints and should be rated for hard/extra-hard usage and must be marked every foot along the length with the code for the type of usage. Extension cords must be grounded 3-prong type.

Classifications of Work Injuries

Work injuries can be classified in a variety of manners, one of which is according the type of accident. The types of accidents are divided into the following categories:

- Struck by (work hit by moving object).
- Caught in, under, between (body part pinched or crushed).
- Struck against (worker collides with stationary object).
- Fall from elevation (fall from a higher to a lower level).
- Falls on same level (incident when a worker loses footing).
- Motor vehicle accidents (motor vehicle crashes on or off of the worksite).
- Overexertion and repetitive trauma (injuries as a result of excessive physical exertion or repetitive patterns of movement).
- Other causes of physical trauma (contact with electric current, radiation, temperature extremes, chemicals, tissue abrasions).

Musculoskeletal Disorders That Can Affect Workers

De Quervain's Disease

It is a musculoskeletal disorder that affects the thumbs. A symptom of the disorder is pain at the base of the thumb and is caused by excessive twisting and gripping. Some of the workers that can be affected by De Quervain's disease are butchers, housekeepers, packers, seamstresses, and cutters.

Trigger Finger

It is a musculoskeletal disorder that affects the index finger. The symptoms of the disorder include difficulty moving the finger and snapping/jerking movements. It is caused by repetitive use of the index fingers. Some of the workers that can be affected by trigger finger are meatpackers, poultry workers, carpenters, and electronic assemblers.

Rotator Cuff Tendinitis

It is a musculoskeletal disorder that affects the shoulders. The symptoms of the disorder include shoulder pain and stiffness. It is caused by frequently working with the hands over the head. Some of the workers that can be affected by rotator cuff tendinitis are power press operators, welders, and assembly line workers.

Tenosynovitis

It is a musculoskeletal disorder that affects the hands and wrists. The symptoms of the disorder include pain and swelling. It is caused by repetitive or forceful hand and wrist motions. Some of the workers that can be affected by tenosynovitis are cake makers, poultry processors, and meat packers.

Raynaud's Syndrome

It is a musculoskeletal disorder that affects the fingers and hands. The symptoms of the disorder include numbness, tingling, ashen skin, and a loss of feeling and control. It is caused by exposure of the hands to vibration. Some of the workers that can be affected by Raynaud's syndrome are chain saw, pneumatic hammer, and gasoline-powered tool operators.

Carpal Tunnel Syndrome

It is a musculoskeletal disorder that affects the fingers and wrists. The symptoms of the disorder include tingling, numbness, severe pain, and loss of strength or sensation in the thumbs, index finger, middle finger, or half of the ring finger. It is caused by repetitive and forceful manual tasks with no time to recover. Some of the workers that can be affected by carpal tunnel syndrome are meat, poultry, or garment workers, upholsterers, assemblers, VDT operators, typists, and cashiers.

Back Disability

It is a musculoskeletal disorder that affects the back. The symptoms of the disorder include lower back pain and shooting pain or numbness in the upper legs. It can be caused by heavy lifting or whole body vibrations. Some of the workers that can be affected by back disability are truck and bus drivers, tractor and subway operators, warehouse workers, nurse's aides, grocery cashiers, and baggage handlers.

Risk Factors

The **risk factors that can cause musculoskeletal disorders** are as follows: awkward postures (postures that put added stress or restrict the flow of blood to joints or muscles), forceful exertions (activities that put higher loads of force on the muscles such as lifting, pushing, or pulling), repetitive motions (motions that are repeated frequently for prolonged periods of time), contact stresses (repeated or continuous contact with hard or sharp objects), vibration (when parts of the body come into contact with a vibrating object), and compression (grasping hard or sharp edges where pressure and restricted blood flow is concentrated on one area of the body). Other workplace conditions that can cause or increase the risks of developing musculoskeletal disorders include cold temperatures, insufficient pauses or rest breaks, machine-paced work, as well as unfamiliar work.

Ergonomics

Ergonomics is the study of how the physical demands of work and the work environment affect the physical well-being of the worker. It is a discipline that focuses on matching the physical abilities of the worker to the job and eliminating/redesigning work practices or processes that put too much strain on workers. The process of developing an ergonomically sound workplace entails designing furniture, equipment, tools, and work processes in such a way that they correspond to both the physical capabilities of the workers and do not cause excessive physical stress or strain. The key to this procedure is having an understanding of the limits of physical stress on the body before injury will occur, as well as particular activities that are high risk for developing musculoskeletal disorders.

VDTs

Visual-display terminal workstation design should focus on ergonomics to prevent injury and reduce stress. The VDT workstation should be positioned for the most appropriate line of sight so that the user doesn't need to swivel or look to the side frequently. OHSA provides a checklist to ensure proper design:

- **Monitors**: Screen should be large enough to easily read and perform tasks and should be adjustable. Docking stations should be available for laptops.
- **Keyboards**: Alternative (ergonomic) keyboards should be available with long enough cords to allow repositioning and adjustable from 22 -30 (sitting) to 36-46.5 inches (standing) from floor and positioned at elbow height. Keyboards without the 10-key keypad should be used if the keypad is rarely used so that the mouse can be positioned closer to the keyboard to prevent joint stress.
- **Keyboard trays:** Should be 22 to 18.3 inches from the floor and adjustable.
- **Desk**: Should be large enough for equipment and supplies. Clearance depth for knees is 17.6 inches and 24 inches for feet. Clearance width is at least 20.8 inches and 20 inches for knee height. Desktops should be matte/non-glare and glass should be avoided because of risk of breakage, glare, and injury.

Specialty Areas

The study of ergonomics has three different **specialty areas**. They are as follows:

- **Human Factors Engineering** (Engineering Psychology): Studies the engineering controls (gauges, warning buzzers, signs, instructions, and controls) that can affect the well-being of the worker as a result of the potential for error in a work process.
- **Anthropometry**: The design of clothing, machines, furniture, and tools with the fit of the worker in mind.
- **Occupational Biometrics**: Studies the effects of work on muscles and other connective tissues and development of musculoskeletal disorders as a result of overexertion of the worker.
- **Work Physiology**: Deals with the ways work affects the cardiovascular system, pulmonary system, and skeletal muscles with the goal of preventing body fatigue.

OSHA Ergonomic Guidelines

The **OSHA ergonomic guidelines** were developed for the meatpacking industry in 1991 with the purpose of giving employers the information necessary to assess the workplace and determine if there are health and safety issues related to ergonomics. Since, they have expanded on guidelines to other work environments where physical stress and overexertion can result in injury to the worker. The guidelines stress that both management support and worker commitment are critical components to a successful ergonomic program. Industries with guidelines currently recommended by OSHA include the following: agriculture, footwear and apparel, baggage handling, beverage delivery, carpet laying, computer workstations, construction, food distribution centers, foundries, furniture manufacturing, healthcare, manufacturing, meatpacking, mining, poultry processing, printing, sewing, and shipyards. OSHA stresses that these are simply guidelines/recommendations, therefore companies cannot be punished for violating these recommendations.

According to the OSHA guidelines, there are six elements of an ergonomic program. They are Management Leadership and Employee Participation, Hazard Information, Job Hazard Analysis and Control, Training, MSD management, Ergonomic Program Evaluation, and Records.

Worksite Analysis

Worksite analysis is an important element of the job hazard analysis within an ergonomic program as outlined by OSHA. It entails the assessment of the workplace to identify working conditions and work processes that are high risk for causing injury to the worker. This includes a thorough analysis of medical records for work-related illness and injury, as well as the detection of activities or aspects of the work environment that are linked to the development of musculoskeletal disorders. Worksite analyses should be conducted at regular intervals so that physical stress and strain can be detected before anyone is injured.

Engineering Control Strategies

Hazard information is another aspect of an ergonomic program as outlined by OSHA. **Engineering control** strategies are considered the most effective way to reduce the stress and strain caused by physical overexertion. This includes the design of the worksite, tools, and work processes. Some of the ways that engineering can control ergonomic-related injuries include using mechanical aids to help a worker move materials or equipment, employing technology to reduce physical exertion, changing the layout of the environment or tool design, and changing the order of operations.

Administrative Control Strategies

Administrative control strategies address work policies and procedures such as the length of a shift, the number of breaks, the number of employees, and the overall pace of a job. It is important to note that administrative control strategies do not remove a workplace hazard; they simply attempt to control it through the institution of relevant policies and procedures. Thus, the key to the effectiveness of any administrative control measures is management enforcement of these policies.

Management Leadership/Employee Participation

Management leadership and employee participation is also an aspect of an ergonomic program as outlined by OSHA. A successful medical management program should include early detection, reporting, and recording of work related illness or injury; an evaluation and referral system that maximizes occupational health resources, a conservative treatment and return to work policy, program assessment/monitoring activities for quality control, and the sufficient equipping of health/medical services (including personnel, equipment, and supplies). Effective health/medical management also includes the execution of periodic walk-throughs by qualified medical personnel. This endures that workplace activities and processes are fully understood and the potentials for the development of musculoskeletal disorders due to physical stressors are more easily identifiable.

Training

Training is an additional aspect of an ergonomic program as outlined by OSHA. It provides both managers and workers with the information needed to assess the workplace for potential ergonomic hazards. As with any health and safety program, education is the most important tool for the prevention of illness and injury. This particularly the case with new workers, equipment, or work processes. The appropriate use of equipment, the implementation of safety protocols, and the early signs and symptoms of musculoskeletal disorders are all a part of an effective ergonomic training program.

Medical Waste Disposal

Medical Waste Disposal Program

A **medical waste program** is designed to develop procedures for handling, containing, storing, and removing any potentially hazardous waste that is produced in a medical setting (in this case, and occupational health unit). Any discarded material that has a potential to be harmful to human health or the environment is classified as hazardous waste. This harm can be due to any of the aspects of the material including its concentration, physical characteristics, chemical composure, or toxicity. A substance need not possess all of these characteristics to be considered hazardous. Any waste disposal program must be based on current federal and state laws, as well as company policy.

Principles and Practices

A medical waste program should include the following **principles and practices:**

- Handling, placement, and labeling of sharps so as to minimize the potential for human contact. This includes the disposal of sharps in the appropriate container and labeling the container with the biohazard symbol.
- Package medical waste for disposal in a minimum of one leak-proof plastic bag that is strong enough to withstand normal handling.
- Placement of medical waste bags inside of a rigid fiberboard box or drum to prevent and contain the leakage of hazardous materials.
- Liquid medical waste should be disposed of in a leak-proof-capped bottle.
- All hazardous waste bags/containers must be labeled with a water-resistant universal biohazard symbol and should be stored in an area with limited/restricted access.
- Medical waste must be treated in the appropriate manner (sterilization, incineration, gas or vapor sterilization, chemical disinfection, thermal inactivation, and irradiation) either in-house or with a company that specializes in its treatment.
- Medical waste should never be stored long-term.

Interdisciplinary Interactions and Collaborations

There are a number of **interdisciplinary interactions and collaborations** that are necessary when developing a medical waste disposal program. Corporate resources should be utilized whenever possible. In addition to corporate resources, there are many valuable resources outside of the company that are typically available. Some of these include local health departments, state health departments, the Environmental Protection Agency (EPA), other occupational health nurses, physicians, and other companies with medical waste disposal programs already implemented. Not only should there be interdisciplinary interactions and consultations during the development stages of a waste disposal program, but also for regular reviews once the program is implemented. This ensures that the program is thorough in its actions, policies, and compliance with regulations.

Roles of Occupational Health Nurse

An **occupational health nurse** has many **roles** in a medical waste disposal program. These roles include the development of medical waste disposal policies and procedures, educating housekeeping staff and first-aid response team members as to medical waste policy and procedures including relevant emergency procedures, educating employees about hazardous waste handling and disposal. It is important to note that, while the occupational health nurse is responsible for organizing and maintaining a medical waste disposal program, the collaboration of many others (from employees to community resources) is a necessary part of an effective waste management program.

Psychophysiologic/Stress

Managing Psychosocial Factors in the Workplace

Psychosocial factors involve both the social and psychological (mental health) aspects of a person's life. There are a number of psychosocial factors that influence an individual's perception their coworkers and job satisfaction. Because work is such a big part of our lives today, job satisfaction can have an impact (both positively and negatively) on our quality of life and social interactions, both inside and outside of the work environment. Thus, it is the responsibility of occupational health personnel to have an understanding of the social and psychological influences within the workforce so that they can adequately manage, educate, and evaluate workers regarding this aspect of workplace health.

Worker Approach and Workplace Approach

There are two basic approaches to **managing psychosocial factors** in the workplace:

- The first is the **worker approach**. This entails providing workers with the appropriate tools to adequately deal with the negative aspects of psychosocial factors. Some typical worker-related services include stress management, employee assistance, and counseling.
- The second approach to managing psychosocial factors is the **workplace approach**. This approach addresses psychosocial factors and stressors by improving the work environment. It is an OSHA recommended way to deal with workplace psychosocial factors because it endeavors to address the stress by removing the stressor.

Elements That Influence Psychosocial Factors in the Workplace

There are a number of **psychosocial factors** that **influence** an individual's perception their coworkers and job satisfaction. The psychosocial factors that affect workers are complex and multifaceted. There is not one single aspect of the work environment that affects it, but many that work together to produce psychosocial hazards. Some of the elements within the workplace that influence psychosocial factors include the structure and characteristics of the workers and work processes; organizational characteristics and culture; work-related interpersonal relationships; the significance of work and the work environment to both the workers and the organization.

Effects of Societal Tensions and Conflicts in the Workplace

As a workplace counselor, the occupational health nurse can help coordinate changes in areas that are causing tension in the workplace. There are many possible **societal tensions and conflicts** that can have an effect on worker relationships. Age, ethnic, and gender discrimination as well as sexual harassment are all potential points of workplace conflicts. Personal conflicts, such as balancing the demands of work and family, can also cause a great deal of tension on workers. These tensions and conflicts must be resolved if both the workplace and employees' personal lives are to remain well balanced and functional.

Psychosocial Hazards in the Workplace

Psychosocial hazards are less concrete and more difficult to define than physical hazards. They are complex and multifaceted with many factors influencing the level of severity. With that being said, there are still several **psychosocial hazards that can be identified as pervasive** in today's work environment. They are as follows:

- **Workplace violence** – An act of aggression that causes harm (physical or psychological) to a worker. Includes threats, harassment, intimidation, stalking, etc. This violence may be lateral (peer-peer) or vertical (between different ranking employees).
- **Mistreatment and harassment** – An act against a worker that results in an unfriendly and threatening work environment. Includes yelling, ridiculing, sexual harassment, etc.
- **Unemployment and underemployment** – Threats to employment security (such as contingent, temporary, and part-time worker) have serious effects on the physical and psychological well-being of the workforce.
- **Shift work** – Evening, night, or rotating shifts.
- **Characteristics of work** – Work overload, underload, role conflict, and role ambiguity.

Assessing Psychosocial Factors in the Workplace

There are two steps in **assessing psychosocial factors** in the workplace:

1. The first is to identify the conditions in the workplace that are potential psychosocial hazards. This step entails reviewing the different jobs and their descriptions; interviewing employees and managers; conducting workplace walk-throughs; and having group discussions that include management, labor representatives, and the workers.
2. The second step, once hazards or stressors have been identified, is to measure the actual stress reaction using subjective and objective techniques. Subjective techniques include self-reports, job satisfaction, and workplace morale. Objective techniques entail analyzing worker data such as turnover rates, absenteeism, and healthcare costs.

CISD

Critical incident stress management (CISM) is a procedure to help people cope with stressful events, such as disasters and traumas, in order to reduce incidence of post-traumatic stress syndrome. **Critical incident stress debriefing (CISD)** includes:

- **Defusing sessions** usually occur very early, sometimes during or immediately after a stressful event, and are used to educate personnel who are actively involved about what to expect over the next few days and to provide guidance in handling feelings and stress.
- **Debriefing sessions** usually follow in one to three days and may be repeated periodically as needed. These sessions may include people who were directly involved as well as those indirectly involved. People are encouraged to express their feelings and emotions about the event. The six phases of debriefing include introduction, fact sharing, discussing feelings, describing symptoms, teaching, and reentry. Critiquing the event or attempting to place blame is not productive as part of the CISM process.
- **Follow-up** is done at the end of the process, usually after about week but this can vary.

Preventing and Controlling Negative Effects of Psychosocial Factors in the Workplace

There are several ways to **prevent and control psychosocial factors** in the workplace. The type of intervention necessary is relative to the type of stressor. Thus, it is important to conduct a thorough analysis of the workplace. Once a stressor has been identified, it is important that the intervention is appropriate and effective. Once the intervention is implemented it should be evaluated for efficacy. Other ways to prevent stress related to psychosocial factors in the workplace is to educate workers, obtain management support and commitment to eliminating stressors, involve the workers in the process of stressor elimination, and secure the resources necessary to develop an effective occupational health program.

Impact of Diagnosable Mental Illnesses on the Workplace

Mental illnesses can have a major impact on the workplace. Today, many mental illnesses are both diagnosable and treatable. Some of the diagnosable mental illnesses that an occupational health nurse may encounter are as follows:

- **Anxiety and depression**: The most common psychiatric disorders in the US.
- **Psychotic disorders**: Not very common, but can greatly affect an individual's capabilities, reasoning, and judgment, thus reducing their functional abilities in society and the workplace.
- **Personality disorders**: More common than psychotic disorders. Affects the ability of an individual to relate to others, thus increasing the possibility of conflicts developing with other workers.

Addressing Employees with Depression

If an employee is showing signs or **depression** (fatigue, loss of energy, loss of appetite, abnormal sleep patterns), it is important to conduct a complete assessment so that the appropriate support and interventions can be suggested. This assessment includes utilizing communication and empathetic listening skills to get the employee to open up, as well as asking questions targeted at depression so as to come to an understanding of the possible reasons for the depressive symptoms. If the depression worsens or if it looks like a person may attempt to harm themselves, referral for immediate intervention is necessary.

Behavioral Indicators of Emotional Distress

As a workplace counselor, the occupational health nurse may have to deal with employees in **emotional distress**. Thus, it is important to have a knowledge and understanding of some of the behavioral indicators of emotional distress. They are as follows:

- Increased or persistent absenteeism, with regular absences on Mondays, Fridays, and after payday.
- Increased fatigue and sleeping with a decrease in the ability to concentrate and complete tasks.
- Increased number of accidents, injuries, or mistakes made at work.
- Decrease in interpersonal relationships with an increase in criticism of others.
- Notable negative changes in mood and/or appearance.
- Physical symptoms of stress such as weight loss, stomach problems, and headache.
- Substance abuse problems.

Occupational Stress

Occupational stress is defined as the harmful physical and emotional reactions to a job when there is a disparity between the job requirements and the abilities of the worker, requirements of the worker, or available resources within the company. Both acute and chronic stress responses can occur:

- **Acute stress responses** describe reactions that have a sudden onset, short duration, and no long-term effects.
- **Chronic stress responses** are responses that have a long duration such that negative physiologic, psychological, or behavioral effects are realized.

There are many different possible causes of occupational stress. They include (but are not limited to) heavy workload, long hours or shift work, repetitive tasks, not enough breaks between tasks or jobs, communication and management styles, work and non-work interpersonal relationships, unclear or disproportionate job responsibilities, anxiety over career development, and poor workplace environmental conditions.

Effects of Stress on Workers

Physiologic, psychological, and behavioral responses can occur when **workers** are subjected to occupational stress. Examples of some of these responses are as follows:

- **Physiologic responses** – Cardiovascular disease, musculoskeletal disorders, gastrointestinal disorders, reduced immune system functioning.
- **Psychological disorders** – Depression, posttraumatic stress disorder, emotional exhaustion, depersonalization, reduced personal accomplishment.
- **Behavioral responses** – Reduced performance, decreased attention, increased distractibility, poor judgment, irritation, self-neglect, interpersonal conflict.

Effects of Stress on Organizations

When there is a high level of stress in the workplace, organizations realize a negative effect that is different but related to the physiologic, psychological, and behavioral responses that a worker experiences. The effects of **stress on organizations** relates to work performance and economic ramifications. When workers are under stress, they are less productive and the quality of work is compromised, resulting is a decrease in overall work performance. There are also economic consequences to occupational stress that are manifested in an increase in workman's compensation claims, increased insurance costs, increased absenteeism and tardiness, and increased worker turnover.

Physical, Psychological, and Behavioral Stress-Related Symptoms and Disorders

Stress is common in our lives today. Quite often, this stress has a direct link to factors and responsibilities in workplace. Because an occupation health program focuses on the health of the workers and prevention of work-related illness and injury, it is important for an occupational health nurse to recognize the different physical, psychological, and behavioral **symptoms** and disorders that are related to stress. They are as follows:

- **Physical**: Fatigue, headache, musculoskeletal disorders, hypertension, heart disease, gastrointestinal problems, and infection.
- **Psychological**: Irritability, anger, depression, apathy, anxiety, worry, and withdrawal.
- **Behavioral**: Smoking, overeating, substance abuse, insomnia, hostility, burnout, and absenteeism.

Workplace Factors That Influence Stress State

The **six workplace factors that influence the stress state** are as follows:

1. **Personal Factors** – Personal factors that include the health of the individual, character traits, coping and communication abilities, and personal morals and values.
2. **Situational/Interpersonal Factors** –Job-specific factors that include the existence of a workplace support system, ability to get along with coworkers, and the way the individual is treated (i.e. respected).
3. **Organizational Factors** – Work-related policies that includes the amount of work and individual is responsible for, the role of the workers in the company, the quality of communication, leadership, and managerial skills in the workplace.
4. **Technological Factors** – Factors associated with technology-based systems that include complicated equipment, job procedure/process design, computers, and communications networks.
5. **Environmental Factors** – Location-specific factors that include the workstation design and ergonomic controls, the amount of light, noise, odors, and number of workers in a given area.
6. **Economic Factors** – Financially based factors that include job protection, pay scale, number and cost of benefits, and an individual's personal standard of living.

Psychophysiologic Hazards Associated with Shift Work

Shift work is work outside of the normal (9am to 5pm) work schedule, such as evenings and nights or 12-hour shifts. Some shift work is rotating; that is, the person changes shifts on a regular schedule, such as every two weeks. Psychophysiologic hazards associated with shift work include:

- Increased incidence of chronic diseases, such as heart disease, GI disorders, metabolic disorders, and obesity as well as some types of cancer.
- Sleep disorders because of decrease in production of melatonin during the night (decreased light exposure) and circadian rhythm disruption. People doing shift work tend to sleep less than those on other schedules and face more interruptions of sleep, leading to sleep deprivation.
- Impaired performance because the ability to concentrate is impacted and reaction time tends to be slower.
- Depression more likely because of disruptions of relationships with other and circadian rhythm disruption.
- Accidents and injuries because people are sleepy or decision-making is impaired. Additionally, less supervision and assistance are often available, so accidents/errors are more likely to occur.

Travel-Related Issues That Impact Psychophysiologic Well-Being of Workers

Many workers are required to **travel for work**, but this can lead to a number of problems:

- **Unproductive time:** While the workload may remain unchanged, working on an airplane or other mode of transportation can be difficult if not impossible, so the worker is often left with too few hours to do too many tasks, and work can pile up.
- **Jet lag:** Travel from one time zone to another can interfere with sleep patterns and result in chronic sleepiness/fatigue, GI upset, and depression.
- **DVT**: Sitting for long periods of time increases the risk of deep vein thrombosis because of stasis.

- **Unplanned/unforeseen occurrences**: Planes may be delayed, luggage lost, connections missed, and meetings delayed, resulting in increased stress and anxiety.
- **Changed routine**: Mealtimes may be different, resulting in hunger or lack of appetite, and time restrictions may result in increased intake of fast food and unhealthy snacks.
- **Family disruption**: The worker may have little time for family or may miss important family milestones (birthdays, holidays, graduations) because of work commitments.

STRESS PREVENTION

The **National Institute for Occupational Safety and Health** has outlined three steps that can help **prevent occupational stress**. They are as follows:

1. **Identify the Problem** - Hold discussion groups; provide employee surveys; evaluate employee opinion of working conditions, stress, health, and fulfillment to identify problem areas and conditions prone to stress development.
2. **Design and Implement Interventions** - Deal with the source of stress by suggesting specific intervention strategies, discussing these interventions with relevant employees, and implementing the interventions.
3. **Evaluate Interventions** - Both short-term and long-term evaluations must be conducted to determine the effectiveness of the implemented interventions. This is accomplished by evaluating employee opinion of working conditions, stress, health, and employee perception of job condition. If problem areas are found, changes should be made, the new interventions implemented, and the entire evaluation process conducted again.

FITNESS FOR DUTY FOR RETURN TO WORK AND JOB READINESS

Fitness for duty is the physical, mental, and emotional ability to carry out required job functions. Candidates for a position may not be required to have a physical exam before hiring, but a preplacement exam may be required before placing the person in a position in order to assure that the person is able to do the necessary work. When assessing fitness for duty, regulations regarding the ADA, FMLA, and EEOC must be considered and the fitness for duty policy must be applied equally to all and based on the specific requirements of the job. If an employee has medical leave under FMLA for a serious personal health problem, then the employer may request a fitness-for-duty certification by a healthcare provider before the employee returns. The employer must issue a designation notice regarding the need for the certification and can include a list of essential job functions that must be addressed in the fit-for-duty certification. The employer can delay the employee's return to work until the certification is received.

EMPLOYEE ASSISTANCE PROGRAMS

An **employee assistance program** (EAP) is part of the benefit package offered employees in many organizations. The purpose of the program is to assist employees with personal or work-related problems that interfere with their ability to carry out their jobs. While EAPs vary, they usually include counselling services and referrals. Supportive services may be available for PTSD, workplace violence, substance (alcohol, drug) abuse, domestic violence, occupational stress, emotional stress, financial issues, legal concerns, and life events (births, deaths, illness, disability). Participation in an employee assistance program is usually voluntary and free of cost (although there may be costs associated with referrals), and participation remains confidential in order to encourage those with problems to take advantage of the program. With some programs, the services are also available to immediate family members. EAPs are available in federal and state agencies as well as in the private sector.

Pre-Employment Screening Process

Pre-employment drug screening is common in the transportation industry (pilots, bus drivers, ambulance drivers) and many other industries because of concerns regarding safety and drug use. Drug screening may be done by obtaining various samples:

- **Blood**: detects present drug use)
- **Urine**: required for federally-mandated screening, detected use varies according to the drug
- **Saliva**: detects use within 2 days.
- **Hair**: detects use within 90 days. 100-120 strands of hair are cut off close to the scalp and collected.

Chain of custody screening documents each step in the collection and testing to reduce the incidence of tampering. Procedure:

1. Identity of donor confirmed.
2. Specimen collected in secure private room and specimen sealed into container in donor's presence, always keeping the sample within view.
3. The chain of custody form is completed by both the donor and lab technician.
4. Specimen is sealed into a transport bag and shipped to laboratory in a manner that does not allow the public access to the specimen with transport records maintained.
5. The specimen should be received by a medical review officer.

Aging as Related to Occupational Psychophysiologic Response/Stress

As the workforce ages and the cost of living remains high, many **aging adults** remain in the workforce but may face psychophysiologic issues:

- **Age discrimination:** Younger workers may view older works as less valuable ("outdated") and show little respect, and older workers often must report to younger supervisors and bosses, resulting in anxiety and stress. Older workers may feel unwanted at work.
- **Chronic illness**: Older workers may have to cope with physical problems (heart disease, diabetes, arthritis, hypertension), which can decrease their stamina and result in fatigue, pain, and other problems.
- **Sick time**: Studies show that older workers tend to take more sick time than younger workers and take longer to recover from illness, impacting their chances for promotion and sometimes causing resentment on the part of other workers.
- **Limitations in physical strength/abilities**: Older workers may require job accommodations or may be unable to carry out work functions, especially in blue-collar jobs.

Impact of Culture on Psychological Response to Work-Related Stress

Cultural differences can affect perceptions of and psychological response to work-related stress. Increasingly international companies pair workers from different cultures, and foreign workers are common in some industries, so recognizing and understanding differences is essential. Workers often have very different ideas about work. For example, some workers may feel that working overtime is simply part of the job while others may refuse to work overtime because doing so impacts their social or family life, resulting in misunderstanding, mistrust, and resentment on both parts. In cultures where people tend to be less direct, negative comments or advice may result in feelings of inadequacy, anger, and confusion. Some may expect that their nonverbal language (expressions, silence) conveys a message as effectively as spoken language, but the nonverbal language may be completely misunderstood by someone of a different culture. Workers in some cultures may express their concerns openly while others may suffer silently. Workers may encounter hostility, especially those with different religions or manners of dress; this can increase anxiety, stress, and resentment.

Disaster

A **disaster** is an event where many people are exposed to hazards that results in injury, death, and damage to property. There are a number of hazards that have the potential to lead to a disaster situation. In general, they can be classified as natural, technological, or caused by human conflict. Some specific examples of each are as follows:

- **Natural**: Firestorms, flood, land shift, tornado, epidemic, earthquake, volcano, hurricane, high winds, blizzard, heat wave.
- **Technological**: Hazmat spills, explosions, utility failure, building collapse, transportation accident, power outage, nuclear accident, dam failure, fire, water loss, ruptured gas main.
- **Human Conflict**: Riots, strikes, suicide bombings, bomb threat, employee violence, mass shootings, equipment sabotage, hostage events, transportation disruption, weapons of mass destruction, computer viruses/worms.

Disaster Management Plans

There are several different **types of disaster management plans**, some more specific than others. They are listed and briefly described below:

- **Emergency Action Plan** – OSHA required, evacuation plans and emergency drills.
- **Business Continuity Plan** – Business operation-specific, aimed at reducing losses and resuming productivity.
- **Risk Management Plan** – Off-site effects of chemical exposures.
- **Emergency Response Plan** – Immediate response to disasters.
- **Contingency Plan** – General, designed to handle events not covered in other plans.
- **Federal Response Plan** – Coordinates federal resources.
- **Spill Prevention, Control, and Countermeasures Plan** – Deals with the prevention, control, and clean-up of oil spills.
- **Mutual Aid Plan** – Plan for shared resources between other companies/firms.
- **Recovery Plan** – Deals with repair and rebuilding post-disaster.
- **Emergency Management Plan** – Plan for healthcare facilities.
- **All-Hazard Disaster Management Plan** – General plan that is not hazard-specific.

Development

There are many different types of disaster management plans. Regardless of the type, however, there are several **basic steps for its development.** To begin with, a planning team must be established that includes representatives from all levels within the organization. The planning team is responsible for putting together a timeline for completion of the plan as well as an estimation of the costs, fees, and resources necessary to complete the plan. Once this is done, an analysis of potential disasters can begin. In this step, potential hazards are identified and vulnerability of the organization to disasters is assessed. A disaster response plan is established that includes the reduction/removal of hazardous situations. The final steps are plan implementation and review. The plan can be tested for efficacy through drills and mock disaster situations. It is critical to review and update the plan yearly.

Stages of Disaster/Emergency Response Within the Workplace

Once a disaster has occurred in the workplace, there are basic **stages of the response process.** They are as follows (in order of operation):

1. Recognition that a disaster has occurred.
2. Notification of management and employees of the disaster.
3. Take steps to guarantee the immediate safety of employees
4. Take steps to guarantee public safety, protection of property, and protection of the environment.

The length of each stage depends on the scope of the disaster and how well previous stages were executed. Because people are the first priority of any disaster/emergency response, if there are any people left in harm's way, property and the environment cannot become a focus of protection.

ICS

The **Incident Command System (ICS)** was developed by the Department of Homeland Security as a part of the National Incident Management System. It is a highly organized, hierarchical disaster management system that focuses on planning and organization, communication and delegation of responsibility, as well as response evaluation so that any disaster/emergency response effort runs as smoothly as possible. An Incident Commander (IC) is established as the person in charge. Safety officers, operations section officers, planning officers, and logistics officers are all appointed. These different officer positions are responsible for reporting back to the IC.

Disaster Recovery Aspect of Disaster Planning and Management

Disaster recovery is the final stage of any disaster response and deals with the actions necessary to return the disaster site to normal. The recovery effort can be divided into two different periods: restoration and reconstruction/replacement:

- The **restoration period** is an immediate recovery step in which the area is made safe, utilities repaired, wreckage removed, and evacuees are allowed to return.
- The **reconstruction/replacement period** is a longer process where the disaster area is rebuilt and returned to its pre-disaster condition, both physically and economically. The reconstruction period can take many years, and is dependent on the degree of damage and availability of resources for reconstruction efforts. As a part of the disaster recovery process, steps should be taken to prevent a recurrence of the disaster in the future.

Terrorism

Terrorism is defined as the use of violence (or threat of violence) to frighten and coerce governments or societies into accepting the instigator's (terrorists) demands. The demands and goals of terrorists are often extreme and focused on areas with high population densities. This means that large companies can become potential targets of a terrorist attack. For this reason, when developing an emergency preparedness/disaster management plan, terrorist attacks should be included as a potential disaster. There are many different possible ways that terrorists can strike. Some examples are weapons of mass destruction, biological agents (i.e. bacteria, viruses, or toxins), nuclear and radiological incidents, incendiary devices, chemicals, and explosive devices.

Safety and Industrial Hygiene Issues

Safety Programs

Safety Programs and Safety Professionals

Since safety is the responsibility of everybody, the best way to prevent an accident is to ensure that the entire workforce is aware of safety and health issues in the workplace. Thus, this is a primary focus of any **safety program**, and training and educating workers on safety issues are critical parts of a safety professional's job. All employees, including workers, managers, and supervisors, should be trained so that they are aware of safety procedures. **Safety personnel** are in charge of designing the safety program, carrying out relevant procedures, and assessing the workplace for compliance and the program for effectiveness. The ultimate goal of a safety program it the prevention of incidents that result in injury or death.

Planning Safety Programs

In 1997, the National Safety Council outlined five steps that safety professionals should take when **planning a safety program**. They are as follows:

1. Work with top officials in designing a health and safety plan. To ensure management commitment to the program, be sure that safety programs are incorporated into the business plan and strategy of the company.
2. Identify and define the safety roles and responsibilities of everyone in the organization. Evaluate employees for compliance with responsibilities.
3. Continually analyze the workplace so that potential hazards are identified. Set priorities and work to continuously improve the work environment.
4. Set goals and strategies for achieving a safe work environment. Implement actions to achieve these goals.
5. Train all employees, including workers, managers, and supervisors so that all are aware of safety procedures.

Policy Components of Effective Safety Programs

The **five basic policy components** that lead to an effective safety program are as follows:

1. A commitment to providing the safest work environment possible. This includes ensuring that the workplace, work processes, tools, and equipment are all designed with safety in mind.
2. A requirement that all occupational injuries or illnesses be reported and steps taken to prevent future occurrences.
3. An explanation to all employees of the hazards and health risks they may be exposed to and ways to minimize the risks.
4. Regularly scheduled workplace safety analyses so that potential hazards can be identified and addressed before accident or injury occurs.
5. Disciplinary action when employees are not in compliance with safety regulations.

Occupational Safety Program

Safety Director

Safety is the responsibility of everyone, and there are many people that play a role in a safety program. Large companies often hire a safety director. The **safety director** is responsible for developing, implementing, and supervising the safety program across all departments within an organization. Some of the responsibilities of a safety director include conducting workplace inspections and accident investigations, maintaining current and accurate records of accident or injury, employee education and training, and hazard identification and control. Because safety should be kept in mind when designing the workplace and work processes, a safety director often works with other departments (such as engineering and purchasing) during planning and development processes.

Line Supervisor

Line supervisors are one part of the entire framework of an occupational safety program. Because they work with both equipment and the workers, they play an important part in maintaining a safety program. They are responsible for a number of things including implementing safe procedures during line operation, ensuring that current equipment meets safety standards and that new equipment is safe and used according to specifications, assessing line workers for compliance with safety standards, and reporting when accidents or injuries that occur. It is important to remember, however, that safety is the responsibility of everyone, not just the line supervisor.

Occupational Health Personnel

Occupational health personnel are one part of the entire framework of an occupational safety program. This includes both the doctors and nurses that work in an occupational health and safety program. While a large part of what they do is provide primary treatment and care for workers injured at the workplace, they also assist the safety director in assessing the workplace for hazards as well as participate in worksite walk-throughs. By recording and reporting data on workplace injuries to the safety director, occupational health personnel play an important role in accident prevention. It is important to remember, however, that safety is the responsibility of everyone, not just the occupational health personnel.

Employees

Safety is the responsibility of everyone, and the **employees** of a company are one part of the entire framework of an occupational safety program. Ultimately, without employee participation, there would be no safety program. Thus, employee participation is essential for any safety program to be considered a success. In order to participate to their fullest, all workers must be adequately trained in safety procedures. This includes training a worker when they are moved to a new job or area within the company, or when a new work process or piece of equipment is introduced to a current job. In either case, workers need to be educated so that they are well aware of the potential hazards and safety procedures for any new job or process. It is also important to emphasize the need to report any unsafe or hazardous conditions to supervisors.

JSA

A **job safety analysis (JSA)** is an important part in maintaining a safe work environment. It is used to assess the work processes for hazards. Because hazards can develop at any time once production begins or equipment/personnel changes, it is necessary to institute a policy for regular inspection/analysis. There are three basic steps to a JSA. The first is to assess a job and break it down into smaller steps for analysis. Next step is hazard identification. This includes the identification of both current and potential hazards that could result in accident or injury. Finally, the work process must be amended to institute a safe job procedure that eliminates the hazard. This can involve a change in the physical work environment, a change in the steps that make up the job procedure, or a reduction in stress or strain (fewer repetitions, slower pace, less lifting).

Root Cause Analysis

Root cause analysis (RCA) is a retrospective attempt to determine the cause of an event or safety issue, often a sentinel event such as an unexpected death, or a cluster of events. Root cause analysis involves interviews, observations, and review of medical records. Often, an extensive questionnaire is completed by the professional doing the RCA, tracing essentially every step in processes and procedures, including (for healthcare patients) every treatment, every medication, and every contact. The focus of the RCA is on systems and processes rather than individuals. How did the system break down? Where did the problem arise? In some cases, there may be one root cause, but in others, the causes may be multiple. The RCA also must include a thorough review of literature to ensure that process improvement plans based on the results of the RCA reflect current best practices. Plans without RCA may be non-productive. If, for example, an infection was caused by contaminated air, process improvement plans to increase disinfection of the room surfaces would not be effective.

Safety Committee

Because safety is the responsibility of everybody, a **workplace safety committee** is one way for the entire workforce to play a part in developing and implementing workplace safety procedures. Ideally, personnel from all departments and levels of the company should be represented in the committee. This ensures that the safety issues and concerns of all are addressed. The overall purpose of a safety committee is the development of a comprehensive health and safety plan. Once this plan has been designed and implemented, the committee is also responsible for regular (usually annual) evaluation and updating of the plan. In order to cover all aspects of safety, a safety committee should be divided into the following eight task groups: safety activities, rules and procedures, inspections and audits, accident investigation, education and training, health and environment, fire and emergency, and housekeeping.

Safety Activity Task Group

A safety activity task group is one of eight task groups that exist within a safety committee (the other seven task groups are rules and procedures, inspections and audits, accident investigation, education and training, health and environment, fire and emergency, and housekeeping).

Specifically, the safety activity task group is responsible for overseeing the entire safety program, making sure that it is complete and effective, and that all employees are adequately informed about safety procedures. This is done through employee evaluations and participation, data analysis, and the cooperation of the other task groups to institute the necessary steps and procedures for plan improvement.

Rule and Procedure Task Group

Specifically, the rule and procedure task group is responsible for assessing the rules and procedures within the workplace and recommending safer ways to execute them. They are responsible for making sure that all personnel (managers, supervisors, and employees) have knowledge about safe ways to perform every job and work process. In keeping with these responsibilities, the rule and procedure task group recommends compliance procedures and assess if they are being followed, develops a safety manual and for distribution to every department, and recommends necessary education and training.

Inspection and Audit Task Group

Specifically, the inspection and audit task group is responsible for conducting inspections to identify current and potential hazards in the workplace. This includes establishing a schedule for regular inspections, developing and executing an efficient and effective procedure for inspection, gathering and analyzing the data collected during inspections, recommending corrective measures for hazards discovered during an inspection, and assessing compliance with those measures.

Accident Investigation Task Group

Specifically, the accident investigation task group is responsible for looking into every workplace accident to determine the cause and ways to prevent a recurrence of the event. They need to investigate and document every accident in a timely manner, review accident reports, discuss accidents with employees so as to prevent a recurrence, gather and report accident data, and maintain a history of accident reports.

Education and Training Task Group

Specifically, the education and training task group is responsible for training employees on hazard identification and prevention. Since safety is the responsibility of everybody at the workplace, this is a critical group for ensuring the entire workforce is capable of acting in this capacity. In keeping with this responsibility, the education and training task group develops and executes training schedules and procedures, and then assesses these procedures to determine their effectiveness. Because it is the goal of this task group to adequately and appropriately train all personnel, it is necessary to keep thorough records of who has and has not been trained, and what types of training they have received.

Health and Environment Task Group

The purpose of dividing a safety committee into task groups is so that the committee adequately covers all aspects of workplace safety. Specifically, the health and environment task group is responsible for coordinating all activities related to health and environmental safety. This includes assessing safety programs and procedures to ensure that relevant health topics are addressed, conducting health risk assessments and providing health hazard reduction recommendations, as well as suggesting necessary health education and promotion activities.

Fire and Emergency Task Group

Specifically, the fire and emergency task group is responsible for designing and implementing procedures to protect personnel, property, and the environment in case of a fire or other emergency situation. To ensure that all personnel know what to do in emergency situations, it is the responsibility of this task group to develop training programs and procedures, conduct all necessary safety and emergency drills (including evacuation procedures), and assess the workplace and safety procedures to establish emergency preparedness.

Housekeeping Task Group

Specifically, the housekeeping task group is responsible for providing the workplace with the appropriate means for maintaining a clean, orderly, and safe environment. This includes assessing the workplace for cleanliness, providing procedures for maintaining a neat and clean environment, managing waste disposal and clean-up procedures, as well as reporting any environment and housekeeping issues or problems that could adversely affect the health and safety of the works to the proper authorities.

Industrial Hygiene

Industrial hygiene, which exists within the field of environmental science, studies hazards in the workplace and the illnesses and negative health effects that these hazards can cause. Some of these hazards include exposure to physical agents, chemical agents, biological agents, as well as work-related stress. The goal of an industrial hygiene program is to "anticipate, recognize, evaluate, and control" workplace hazards. Because a primary focus of an industrial hygiene program is anticipation and prevention, it can be described as a risk management approach to health and safety, with the overarching goal being to protect the health and safety of the workforce, as well as the community.

Industrial Hygienist

The American Industrial Hygiene Association (AIHA) defines the job of the **industrial hygienist** as follows:

- Anticipate, and therefore prevent, potential workplace hazards.
- Recognize work processes and the stresses associated with them; understand how these processes and stresses can affect the well-being of the workforce and/or community.
- Evaluate, quantitatively whenever possible, the degree to which work processes and stresses negatively affect the health and well-being of the workforce and/or community.
- Suggest necessary steps to eliminate, control, or reduce the negative effects of work processes or stresses with the goal of improving the health and well-being of the workforce and/or community.

Industrial Hygiene Program

Role of Occupational Health Nurse

In large companies, there is sometimes an industrial hygienist on staff. If this is the case, it is the responsibility of the **occupational health nurse** to work with the industrial hygienist in developing an effective risk management program to eliminate workplace hazards. It is often the case, however, that a company does not have a hygienist on staff. In these instances, the occupational health nurse fulfills the role of hygienist by working to "anticipate, recognize, evaluate, and control" workplace hazards. When necessary, a certified industrial hygienist should be consulted to ensure that all potential workplace hazards are addressed.

Hazard Anticipation

Hazard anticipation is the most effective way to prevent workplace hazards and is the first step in implementing an industrial hygiene program. It involves a careful analysis of work processes so that any and all potential hazards can be recognized and any worker exposures can be assessed. Because it is the responsibility of the industrial hygienist to identify hazards before they cause harm, it is important that they are consulted during the planning and implementation phases of developing new processes or technology.

Hazard Recognition

Hazard recognition works hand-in-hand with hazard anticipation, and an industrial hygienist must be able to recognize and identify potential environmental hazards in the workplace. The process of recognition involves the knowledge and understanding of jobs, work processes, and information about toxic chemicals in use. This is gathered through site walk-throughs, environmental sampling, and looking into worker complaints.

Work Process Evaluation

By executing a **comprehensive work process evaluation** when an industrial program is introduced, at the start of new work processes/equipment use, and at various other points in time, an industrial hygienist is able to anticipate and prevent work-related exposures to hazardous conditions. An industrial hygienist must have the knowledge, experience, and resources to be able to successfully complete a work process evaluation.

Information to Be Familiar With

Work process evaluation is a major part of the hazard recognition aspect of an industrial hygiene program. It provides an industrial hygienist with relevant information about the many aspects of the different work processes within the workplace. This information is then used to anticipate and prevent potential workplace hazards. In order to successfully complete a work process evaluation, an **industrial hygienist must become familiar with each of the following**:

- Any work processes and the potential exposures related to these processes.
- Information about physical facilities and environment.
- All chemicals used in work processes including by-products.
- An understanding of the health and environmental hazards related to each chemical used.
- An understanding of the jobs and responsibilities of all workers.
- Knowledge of any workplace control measures currently in place.
- Knowledge of the overall health of workers related to each work process.
- Information gathered from any previous work process evaluations.
- Any additional/new hazards related to a work process.

SDS's

SDS (formerly MSDS) is an acronym that stands for **Safety Data Sheet.** It is a document that is prepared by the manufacturer of a product that provides information regarding the chemical content, chemical properties, and any potential hazards associated with the materials contained in the product, as well as recommendations for safe handling and use of the product. All companies are required by law (U.S. Department of Agriculture, 1987) to keep on hand an SDS for each hazardous chemical on the property. The use of SDS's is an important part of the work process evaluation protocol. It is the responsibility of the industrial hygienist to keep an updated list of all hazardous chemicals used in the workplace. SDSs can aid in compilation of this information. It is important to note, however, that SDS's can sometimes be out of date or incomplete, so it is critical that the industrial hygienist be familiar with and use additional resources.

The **OSHA Hazard Communication Standard** (29CFR 1910-1200 [g]) requires that certain information be included in an SDS. This information is as follows:

- Name of the material as listed on the label.
- Chemical and common names of every ingredient that is a health hazard.
- Physical and chemical characteristics of every hazardous ingredient.
- Physical hazards of chemicals.
- Health hazards of chemicals (including signs and symptoms of exposure, as well as health conditions that can be made worse by exposure).
- Primary routes of entry.
- Exposure limits.
- Carcinogenic status.
- Precautions for safe handling.
- Necessary control measures.
- Emergency and first-aid procedures.
- Date of preparation of SDS.
- Contact information of all parties responsible for development and distribution of SDS.

Common Hazards of Work Processes

A full understanding of the work processes involved in getting a job done is necessary if an industrial hygienist is to recognize the potential health and environmental hazards associated with a job. The **hazards related to common work processes** are as follows:

- **Abrasive Blasting**: Silica and metal dust.
- **Cosmetology**: Chemical exposures.
- **Farming**: Pesticide exposures, heat exposures, heavy lifting, hazardous equipment.
- **Grinding, Polishing, and Buffing**: Inhalation of toxic dusts from metals and abrasives.
- **Painting**: Inhalation of solvents as mists or vapors.
- **Meat Wrapping**: Lifting, standing, repetitive motion, fume exposure from wrap.
- **Welding**: Inhalation of metal fumes, toxic gases, materials.

Hazard Evaluation

Importance of Hazard Evaluation

Industrial hygiene is an important aspect of an occupational health and safety program, so it is critical that program personnel are well trained in the steps of hazard anticipation, recognition, evaluation, and control. After a hazard has been identified, it must go through **the hazard evaluation process.** This is the process that assesses the characteristics and extent of the hazard, as well as the source and route of exposure. When evaluating the extent of the hazard, it is necessary to measure the level of exposure. This is accomplished using hazard-specific tools. For example, air sampling is used for particles, gases, and vapors that can be inhaled; skin wipes measure the amount of physical contact with a substance; and noise dosimeters record noise levels. Using these measurements, worker dose is calculated.

Identifying Potential/Actual Hazards

There are several things that should be taken into consideration in the evaluation process. **Identifying the potential/actual hazards** is one of them. All of the agents or factors that have the potential to cause illness or injury must be identified and classified. This includes biological, chemical, enviromechanical, physical, and psychosocial agents. This process breaks down the hazards into groups, which allows for ease of evaluation. Both actual and potential hazards should be included in this process to ensure that nothing is overlooked.

Identifying When and Where Exposure Occurred

It is important to know both the **location as well as the magnitude of the exposure.** Additional information that should be gathered includes the work process involved, the area/department of the exposure, and the weather/temperature at the time of the exposure. This information is important in identifying problem areas within the workplace.

Identifying Exposed Workers and Means of Exposure

Since the goal of any industrial hygiene program is to eliminate, control, or reduce the incidences of illness or injury due to exposure to environmental hazards, **awareness of exposure**, as well as compliance with **safety protocols at the time of exposure** are critical. In many cases, it is not just the workers directly involved with the work process that are at risk, but others in close proximity to where the exposure occurred.

Identifying Evidence of Exposure

Identifying evidence of exposure involves identifying noticeable physical signs of exposure such as the appearance of smoke, dust, broken machinery, or slippery floors. It also entails studying and prior environmental or health surveys and worker health complaints with current conditions. Of particular concern are reports of coughing, shortness of breath, headaches, dizziness, skin rash, anorexia, fatigue, eye irritation, and numbness/tingling of extremities. These are the most common physical signs and symptoms of exposure. Knowledge and understanding of work-related illness or injury may be necessary in identifying a hazardous exposure in the event of a lack of any obvious physical signs.

Identifying Efficacy of Control Measures

Identifying the **efficacy of control measures** is another consideration in the evaluation process. In many cases, when a hazard is identified, control measures (such as ventilation systems or personal protective equipment) are already in place. It is in these instances that the control measures must be assessed for appropriateness for the identified hazard and, if considered appropriate, effectiveness in controlling it. If equipment is defective or deemed inappropriate for the identified hazard, new measures should be instituted.

Threshold Limit in an Industrial Hygiene Program

Threshold limit is a part of the dose-response relationship. Dose-response describes the correlation between the dose of a chemical and the amount of effect that is realized. Threshold limit describes the dose at which a noticeable effect is realized. Any dose less than this limit produces no measurable effect. It should be understood that, although threshold limit values (TLV's) are used to determine the maximum tolerable level of exposure, they are not always correct. These values are based on toxicity and epidemiological studies, many of which are based on animal experiments that are then extrapolated to humans. So, while they do provide useful information, they do not always translate well to human populations. Because of this, worker exposures should always be kept to the lowest possible dose, and eliminated altogether whenever possible.

There are three ways that **threshold limits are categorized** by the American Conference of Governmental Industrial Hygienists (ACGIH). They are as follows:

1. **Threshold limit value-time weighted average (TLV-TWA):** The time weighted average concentration that all workers are exposed to during a normal workweek (8hrs/day, 40hrs/week) and to which no negative effects are observed. This is a typical, consistently repeated exposure that produces no noticeable harm workers.
2. **Threshold limit value-short term exposure limit (TLV-STEL):** Still within daily TLV-TWA levels, this is the concentration that workers can be exposed to continuously over a short period of time where no noticeable negative effects are observed.
3. **Threshold limit value-ceiling (TLV-C):** This is the concentration that is considered the threshold limit. It is the exposure at which noticeable and measurable negative effects are realized. This limit should never be surpassed.

Permissible Exposure Limits

Worker exposures should always be kept to the lowest possible dose, and eliminated altogether whenever possible. To facilitate the understanding of what is considered an acceptable exposure, the Occupational Safety and Health Administration has developed **permissible exposure limits (PEL's)** for chemicals in the workplace. These limits are based on the threshold limit values (TLV's) developed by the American Conference of Governmental Industrial Hygienists (ACGIH). However, while TLV's are continuously updated, PEL's are often not. Thus, TLV's may be a safer, more accurate way to determine exposure limits. Recommended exposure limits (REL's) are published by the National Institute for Occupational Safety and Health (NIOSH). These are the time weighted average concentrations for up to a 10-hour workday of a 40-hour workweek. Occupational health and safety nurses need to be familiar with each of these lists, but should consult with a trained industrial hygienist for complete understanding and application in the workplace.

HIERARCHY OF CONTROLS

According to NIOSH, the **hierarchy of controls** is the basis for controlling exposure to workplace hazards:

- **Elimination:** Eliminate hazard, change practice. This is the most effective but often the most expensive or most difficult to achieve.
- **Substitution:** Substitute to reduce hazard, such as using a different piece of equipment or process or different chemical.
- **Engineering controls:** Use of shields, barriers, ventilation hoods, guard rails, soundproofing, air conditioning, equipment guards.
- **Administrative controls:** Providing signage, training, adjusted work schedule, rest periods.
- **PPE:** Helmets, safety glasses, gloves, gowns, respirators, face shields. This is the least effective and often indicates the inability to carry out adequate controls at a higher level.

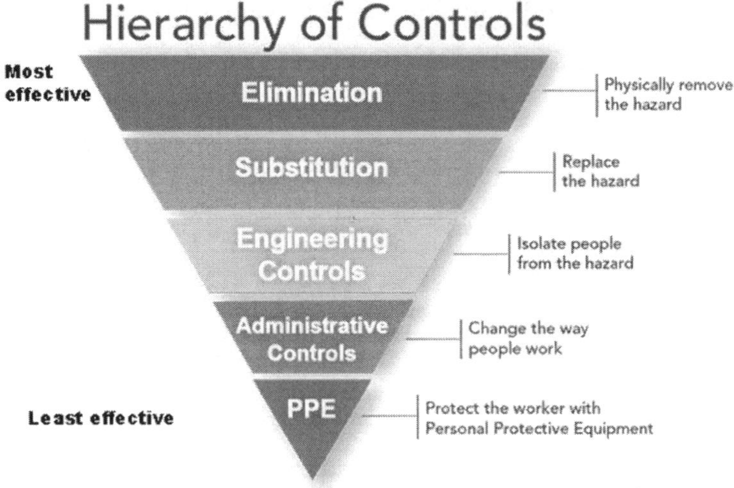

SOURCES OF INFORMATION DICTATING CLASSIFICATION OF A SUBSTANCE OR PROCESS AS A HAZARD

There are three **sources of information** that dictate the **classification of a substance or process as a hazard.** They are as follows:

1. **Scientific literature and exposure limit guides**. Commonly used exposure limit guides are the threshold limit values (TLV's), a set of standards that are established, modified and published yearly by the American Conference of Governmental Industrial Hygienists (ACGIH).
2. **Legal requirements** established by OSHA, as well as federal, state, and local regulations.
3. **Data gathered from worker evaluations**. These should be conducted by healthcare professionals experienced in occupational health and safety issues. In addition to the physical examination of the worker, these evaluations should include work process assessment, worksite assessment, biological sampling, and environmental sampling.

Indoor Air Quality/Radon

Indoor air quality refers to factors in the environmental air that may affect the health or wellbeing of the worker. While OSHA does not have air quality standards, it does provide guidelines. Air quality includes:

- **Ventilation**: Stuffy, poorly-ventilated workplaces may cause headaches, asthma, upper respiratory infections, fatigue. Testing includes air flow and heating and air conditioning systems. Air should be checked for carbon dioxide levels and radon (which can accumulate in buildings) as radon is carcinogenic and can cause lung cancer.
- **Temperature**: Cold or hot environments may cause cold/heat stress as well as shortness of breath, fatigue, general discomfort, and dehydration. Temperatures should be checked in various places in the workplace and at different times of day, including when equipment is in use.
- **Humidity**: Humidity levels should be checked and visual examination made to determine if there is standing water or leakage that may cause water damage, increased humidity, and mold.
- **Hazardous mold/chemicals/gases:** Testing for mold, formaldehyde (a carcinogen found in furniture and building materials), and volatile organic compounds (which can develop from building materials) should be carried out. People exposed to environmental hazards may develop respiratory problems, headache, fatigue, and allergic reactions.

Quantifying Exposures

Sampling Methods

To identify if an exposure event has occurred, an industrial hygienist, or qualified occupational health official, must use the appropriate detecting and **sampling methods** and devices. There are two ways to quantify the level of exposure to gases and vapors. The first is integrated sampling, and the second is grab sampling.

Integrated sampling collects contaminants in the air by a system of moving a known volume of air through a filter over a specific period of time. An average level of exposure is calculated by analyzing the sample on the filter. In order to get an accurate reading of contaminants throughout the day, it is necessary to conduct integrated sampling procedures throughout the entire day.

- When the air is physically forced through the filter using a sampling pump, it is referred to as **active sampling**. Most integrated sampling techniques used and published by OSHA and NIOSH use active sampling techniques.
- When air movement through the filter is not mechanically forced through the filter, but allowed to pass through at natural rates (such as diffusion), it is referred to as **passive sampling**. Passive sampling techniques are utilized in most commercial integrated samplers.

Grab sampling uses a container to collect a sample of air, and then this sample is analyzed for concentration of contaminants. Because this is an instant measurement that provides information about a single point in time, it is not the best technique to use for assessing exposure levels throughout the day. However, if one wants to determine actual contaminant levels at a time when it is known that levels are high, grab sampling it the method of choice.

Skin Contact Exposures and Noise Exposures

Exposure to liquid chemicals typically occurs through the skin. To assess the amount of contamination in the case of skin contact exposure, cloth patches or wipe sampling is used.

When it is a **noise exposure**, sound level meters are used. Either a meter that takes a general reading of the environment, or noise dosimeters that are placed near a worker's ear are employed. Of the two, noise dosimeters are preferred because they give a much more accurate reading of the level of exposure that the individual has experienced.

Direct-Reading Instruments

Direct-reading instruments, also called real-time monitors, are used in identifying and computing exposure levels for gases, vapors, and aerosols. These instruments allow occupational health personnel to analyze air contaminants in the field, allowing them to do away with the need for laboratory analysis. It is an extremely efficient means of analysis because it only takes a few minutes to take a reading and get results. The only drawback is the fact that there is not one direct-read instrument available for detecting and measuring all types of gases, vapors, and aerosols. Thus, it is necessary to have all of the instruments available for the different types of contaminants anticipated in the workplace.

Direct-Reading Instruments for Gases

Commonly used **direct-reading instruments for gases and vapors**, as well as the types of substances they analyze, are as follows:

- Combustible Gas Detectors- Combustible gases vapors.
- Colorimetric Detectors- Vapors such as formaldehyde, hydrogen sulfide, sulfur dioxide, toluene diisocyanate.
- Electrochemical Sensors- Carbon monoxide, nitric oxide, nitrogen dioxide, hydrogen sulfide, sulfur dioxide.
- Infrared Gas Analyzers- Organic and inorganic gases and vapors.
- Metal Oxide Sensors- Hydrogen sulfide, nitro, anime, alcohol, and halogenated hydrocarbons.
- Thermal Conductivity Sensors- Carbon monoxide, carbon dioxide, nitrogen, oxygen, methane, ethane, propane, butane.
- Portable Gas Chromatographs- Organic and inorganic gases and vapors.
- Electron Capture Detector- Halogenated hydrocarbons, nitrous oxide, and compounds containing cyano or nitro groups.
- Flame Ionization Detectors- Organic compounds including aliphatic and aromatic hydrocarbons, ketones, alcohols, and halogenated hydrocarbons.
- Photoionization Detectors- Most organic compounds, especially aromatic compounds.

Determining Acceptable Levels from Exposure Measurements

It is necessary to take into consideration all of the possible routes and time-weighted values of exposure. To determine if the exposure is within acceptable levels, **measurements** must be compared with current standards and guides. To ensure the accurate interpretation of results and understanding of all possible negative health effects, it is necessary to consult any relevant experts (such as the industrial hygienist, occupational health nurse, and consulting physician).

Reducing Workplace Hazards

Instituting Control Measures to Reduce Identified Workplace Hazards

When an occupational hazard is identified and evaluated, a plan of action must be put into place to ensure the remediation of the problem. The following are some of the different ways that **control measures** can be applied so as to reduce the number of workplace hazards:

- Control measures should take into consideration things like the type of hazard, the work processes involved, the number of employees affected, possible routes of exposure, and control methods that are available.
- Using equipment redesign, preventative maintenance, and equipment modification, hazards should be eliminated whenever possible.
- Whenever possible, engineering controls should be employed to eliminate or reduce hazards.
- Control measures should be put into place that limit hazards due to noise, radiation, lightening, heat and vibration, employee work practices should be altered as necessary to eliminate exposures.
- Proper personal protective equipment should be available.
- Educate employees so they understand the potential hazards in the workplace and know how to minimize potential exposures.

Risk Reduction Approaches to Controlling Occupational Health Hazards

Elimination/Substitution

Elimination or substitution of the hazard is one approach to risk reduction. It entails changing either the work process, or the materials used to complete the process, to something that eliminates or reduces the risk of illness or injury. Any elimination or substitution must still ensure that the job can proceed safely. One must be certain the changes to the work process do not compromise worker health or safety. The substitution of one hazard for a lesser, but still hazardous material is considered an unacceptable approach to risk management.

Isolation and Containment

Isolation and containment of the hazard is one approach to risk reduction. It entails physically removing the hazard and containing it so that is away from workers, therefore eliminating the chance for exposure. The containment process usually consists of placing a physical barrier between workers and the hazard. An example of such a barrier is a wall in an effort to reduced exposure to hazardous noise levels, or a plastic container to house needles/sharps.

Engineering Controls

Engineering controls are considered the most effective approach to risk management. It entails the use of engineers to physically change the work environment or work processes by designing and installing new work processes or systems that eliminate the risk of exposure. One typical use of engineering controls in the workplace is the installation of a ventilation system that confines and eliminates dangerous fumes from the work environment.

Work Practice Controls

Work practice controls entail educating management and workers so that all are aware of safe work practices, potential hazards, and ways to reduce exposure. The efficacy of any occupational health or industrial hygiene program is only as good as the workers that conform to safety practices and procedures. Some examples of typical education programs include proper hygiene, safe handling procedures, and good housekeeping.

Administrative Controls

The rotation of workers off a job, the institution of necessary brakes, the reduction of the number of repetitions, and the shortening of the length of work shifts are just a few ways that **administrate controls** can be employed. It is important to understand, however, that administrative controls do not eliminate a hazard; they simply manage and reduce the risk. Administrative controls are ineffective without proper management and oversight.

Personal Protection

Typical **personal protection equipment** includes protective clothing, gloves, head protection, earplugs, goggles and safety glasses, safety shoes, and barrier creams. Worker understanding and compliance with the proper use of protective equipment is an important aspect of the efficacy of personal protection as a means to reduce risk. It is important to understand, however, that the use of personal protection does not eliminate a hazard; it simply manages and reduces the risk. Personal protection equipment becomes ineffective without proper education and compliance.

Safety

Worksite Assessment

Company's Mission

Although a **business's mission** usually does not specifically address health and safety issues, (it deals instead with financial and production issues), it is applied to an occupational health program in the commitment of personnel and resources. In order to conduct a thorough worksite assessment, appropriately trained health personnel need to be available. If, during a worksite assessment, health and safety hazards are discovered, time and resources need to be allocated to remediation activities. Thus, any worksite assessment is only as effective as the company's commitment to the assessment and remediation process.

Management Commitment

Without the cooperation of management, any worksite assessment would be useless. **Management cooperation** is necessary if resources are to be allocated to health personnel so that a worksite assessment can be conducted. This includes providing the equipment, tools, and personnel necessary to conduct an assessment, as well as the materials necessary for the remediation process. If management understands the importance of an occupational health and safety program and remains committed to providing the best possible work environment for employees, then a worksite assessment has the potential to be a useful tool for the occupational health nurse.

Collecting Demographic Information

Demographic information provides insight into the characteristics of a segment of the population. Within the scope of a worksite assessment, the segment of the population under scrutiny is the workforce, and the information included is the number of employees and how they break down into categories by age, sex, ethnicity, department, job title, job responsibilities, and shifts worked. Collecting this information along with accident and illness data can point to problem areas and trends within the workplace.

Without this information, a worksite assessment would not provide the most complete picture of worksite health and safety. All of this information allows the occupational health professional to conduct a well-informed, and therefore effective, worksite assessment.

Dictionary of Occupational Titles

The **"Dictionary of Occupational Titles"** is a resource provided by the United States Department of Labor (1995) that contains standardized occupational information and definitions for over 20,000 jobs. The information includes an occupational category, division, and group, as well as information about the function of the workers and job titles within a category. This information is very useful when conducting a worksite assessment because it provides insight into different jobs so that the occupational health nurse can better understand the workforce. It is a valuable resource for the background information necessary when completing a worksite assessment survey.

Program Review

While the primary purpose of a worksite assessment is to understand and identify workplace hazards and ways to eliminate them, there is also a need to review the health and safety programs that are already in place. A **program review** analyzes current health and safety programs and assesses their ability to meet the needs of workers for which they were designed. It also must be determined if the programs fit the health and safety goals of the organization. This review should be done on a regular basis and any time it is determined that the needs of the workforce have changed or new equipment/technology is introduced.

Review of Program Compliance

Examples of mandated programs include hearing conservation against noise; eye protection against flying objects and chemical exposure; respiratory protection against airborne agents such as lead, silica, asbestos, cotton, and solvent vapor; as well as lock out/tag out safety procedures. If personnel or the organization as a whole are found to be **out of compliance** with mandatory health and safety programs, immediate rectification in the form of administrative controls, engineering controls, and education and counseling is necessary.

Examining and Analyzing Records

While the primary purpose of a worksite assessment is to understand and identify workplace hazards and ways to eliminate them, there is also a need to review the health and safety programs that are already in place. One way to do this is by **examining and analyzing health and safety records.** Some of the records that should be reviewed include written reports, logs, sampling data, health and exposure records, and insurance data. This review should be conducted prior to doing a worksite walk-through so that the occupational health nurse can have a better understanding of relevant illness and injury issues in the workplace. It can also provide insight into any departments, work processes, or particular shifts that appear to increase the likelihood of illness or injury. All of this information allows the occupational health professional to conduct a well-informed, and therefore effective, worksite assessment.

Standard Industrial Classification System

The **Standard Industrial Classification (SIC) system** was developed by the U.S. Office of Management and Budget in 1987. It categorizes United States industries by the type of work they do with the purpose of providing an organized system of classifying statistical information about industry so that is can be used to research and trend analysis. The primary sources of this information are various agencies, associations, and research organizations. The information is divided into different divisions, and within each division into a major group, industry group, and industry code. The structure of the classification system allows for the analysis of the data within a division or group. Data can also be categorized based on work-related illnesses and injuries, thus making SIC codes a useful tool in estimating hazards/risks specific to a particular industry. All of this information allows the occupational health professional to conduct a well-informed, and therefore effective, worksite assessment.

The Standard Industrial Classification (SIC) system covers a variety of **economic activities**. They are as follows: agriculture, forestry, fishing, hunting, trapping, mining, construction, manufacturing, transportation, communications, utilities (electric, gas, sanitation), wholesale trade, retail trade, finance, insurance, real estate, personal, business professional, repair, recreation, services, public administration. These economic activities are broken up into major industrial divisions and given a code. Different workplaces and activities are categorized and given an industry code based on the type of manufactured goods or services offered.

Understanding Work Processes, Materials, and Products

Resource books and technical publications provide information about the hazards inherent to different jobs and work processes. National Institute for Occupational Safety and Health (NIOSH) criteria documents and Safety Data Sheets (SDS) can also provide necessary information about the products, chemicals and by-products used/produced in work processes. All of this information allows the occupational health professional to conduct a well-informed, and therefore effective, worksite assessment.

Knowing and Understanding Raw Materials Used in Work Processes

A complete list of **every chemical and raw material**, as well as their intermediates and by-products, must be obtained and carefully reviewed for potential hazards. The products produced by work processes must also be analyzed for potential to cause harm. Because even low doses of a substance can have the potential to cause harm, all materials must be review regardless of the quantity used. When reviewing the materials used in a work process, how they are being used and the conditions of the environment (closed space, well-ventilated, skin contact, etc.) must be considered because this can greatly affect a substance's toxicity. All of this information allows the occupational health professional to conduct a well-informed, and therefore effective, worksite assessment.

Worksite Assessment Survey

Reviewing Maps

Maps that detail the **layout of the workplace** should always be reviewed prior to conducting a worksite assessment survey so that the person conducting the assessment is familiar with the worksite and can identify operations and specific work areas that have a high risk of resulting in illness or injury (such as repetitive operations and exposure to chemical or physical agents connected to particular work processes). All of this information allows the occupational health professional to conduct a well-informed, and therefore effective, worksite assessment.

Work Process Flow Sheets

The **work process flow sheet** details each step of a work process from start to finish. Some of the details that should be included are any raw materials used, how materials are processed, the equipment and tools that are used, anything that is produced by the process (including byproducts). How byproducts are contained and removed should also be noted. A flow sheet must be created for each and every work process and submitted to the occupational health department/personnel. Work process flow sheets should always be reviewed prior to conducting a worksite assessment survey so that the person conducting the assessment is familiar with the worksite and can identify operations and specific work areas that have a high risk of resulting in illness or injury.

Understanding Workers' Jobs and Associated Activities

In order to identify potential or actual hazards in the workplace, the occupational health nurse must have a thorough understanding of the **different jobs (and their responsibilities) within the workplace**. While a formal job description often contains much of this information, it is still necessary to interview the workers regarding the work that they do. In this way, information gaps or incorrect information can be corrected so as to obtain the most complete and accurate job description possible. All of this information allows the occupational health professional to conduct a well-informed, and therefore effective, worksite assessment.

Job Hazard Analysis

A **job hazard analysis** (also referred to as job safety analysis) is used to find hazardous working conditions that may have been overlooked, could develop once production begins, or may arise with changes in personnel or procedures. A job hazard analysis looks at the safety of a particular job, while a worksite assessment survey looks at the safety of the worksite as a whole. So, while the latter is a broader investigation, the former can provide the necessary detail to ensure a safe working environment. It is best to perform a job hazard analysis as a team (that includes employee participation) and directly observe workers in their environment doing their job. Videotaping can also be employed as a means to capturing the job performance for step-by-step review at another time.

Importance of Familiarity with Work Process Control Measures

Control measures provide concrete steps for controlling an identified hazard. Examples of typical control measures include exhaust fans, ventilation, isolation, shielding, protective clothing, and respiratory equipment. Because new employees, new information, or equipment can make current control measures obsolete or diminish their effectiveness, it is important to current control measures to be sure they are operating as intended. If necessary, suggestions for new control measures should be made that take into consideration new hazards.

Worksite Walk-Through Survey

Goals

When conducting a **worksite walk-through survey**, the occupational health professional tours the worksite during production to observe and gather health and safety information. Specifically, the **five goals** of a worksite walk-through survey are as follows:

1. Recognize and quantify both potential and actual hazards in the workplace by observing workers on the job.
2. Evaluate compliance with occupational health and safety standards.
3. Analyze health and safety policies and programs for successful implementation.
4. Look into complaints of exposure and verify actual exposures.
5. Assess engineering controls for their effectiveness in the remediation of known hazards.

General and Compliance-Related

There are two types of walk-through surveys: general and compliance-related:

- A **general walk-through survey** looks at the operations and procedures at the worksite in an effort to assess work processes for safety, get an idea of baseline exposures to potentially hazardous materials, and identify the physical stresses associated with particular work processes.
- **Compliance-related walk-through surveys** are conducted to determine if management and workers are following mandatory safety procedures (such as OSHA regulations).

Steps

There are four parts to **conducting a worksite walk-through survey**:

1. The first thing to do is to determine the overall purpose of the survey. Is it a comprehensive survey, or a compliance survey? Are certain aspects of the work environment the focus (such as exposure to specific agents or the effectiveness of engineering controls)?
2. Once the purpose has been determined, the second step is to become familiar with worksite operations. This way, the person conducting the survey has an understanding of the chemical agents and physical stresses that are entailed in a job and potential problem areas can be identified.
3. The third step is to prepare for the walk-through by having all necessary supplies available.
4. The final step is to actually conduct the inspection.

All four steps are essential if the occupational health professional is to conduct a well-informed, and therefore effective, worksite walk-through survey.

Becoming Familiar with Worksite Operations

Becoming familiar with **worksite operations** is an important step in preparing for and conducting a worksite walk-through survey. It provides the individual conducting the survey with the information necessary to identify potential problem areas that can be looked into more thoroughly during the survey. Some of the activities included in the familiarization step include examining floor plans, work process flow sheets, and job descriptions; evaluating materials and chemicals used in the workplace; reviewing any relevant health information; and investigating any administrative or engineering controls already in place.

Preparation

Preparing for a walk-through survey by **obtaining necessary supplies** is an important step in the process. Without the appropriate supplies, a survey can become useless because the person conducting it is unable to gather the necessary information. Thus, when considering what equipment is needed, the following must be assessed:

- The presence of gases, vapors, fumes, dusts.
- The need for additional lighting.
- The type of equipment that will be inspected (i.e. boilers, pots, tanks, piping, and hosing).
- Any containers that will require inspection.
- The presence of hazardous supplies (i.e. flammables, explosives, gases, acids, and chemicals).

Inspection Process

The following are the **steps that should be completed during the actual inspection portion of a walk-through survey**:

1. Decide ahead of time which agents require evaluation.
2. Use all of the necessary personal protective equipment.
3. Obtain a sample of the agents under investigation for further testing.
4. Investigate the presence of clearly marked fire exits.
5. Inspect storage areas, equipment, machinery, tools, and electrical equipment for correct and safe operation.
6. Observe compliance to safety regulations.
7. Note housekeeping procedures in all areas being investigated.

Industry Worksite Checklist

An **industry worksite checklist** is a way to organize the aspects of the worksite that are being investigated so that a walk-through can be done systematically and thoroughly. It is also a way to categorize the data that is going to be collected so that when the time comes for analysis, the process is organized and efficient. It is important, however, that the walk-through is not strictly limited to the checklist. It is possible that new environmental safety issues not on the checklist can come to light during the inspection. This can be due to employees, equipment, processes, or environmental conditions that are different from the previous walk-through survey. It is imperative that the person conducting the walk-through be able to recognize the need to inspect aspects of the workplace that were not initially a part of the survey.

Qualitative Evaluation

When conducting a walk-through survey, there are two ways that the worksite can be evaluated: qualitatively and quantitatively. **Qualitative evaluation** relies on the ability of an experienced occupational health professional to detect and assess the scope of a chemical or physical exposure without the use of measuring/assessment tools. It makes use of the knowledge and skills of an individual to examine and evaluate environmental health and safety issues. Qualitative evaluation is useful when tools are not available to quantify a hazard either because the timing of the hazardous situation prohibits the use of measurement devices or because there is no tool in existence to quantify the hazard under investigation. Examples of qualitative evaluation are the visual presence or absence of a substance, the overall condition of equipment, and the degree of compliance to safety policies and procedures.

Quantitative Measurements

Quantitative evaluation involves the use of precise equipment to identify and measure the actual levels of exposure to a hazardous substance. The collected data must first be analyzed before it can be applied to adapting or altering health and safety policies and procedures. Quantitative measurements are an important aspect of a worksite walk-through survey because they provide the data necessary to support a hypothesis. Appropriate use and regular calibration of equipment is necessary for accurate measurements.

Best Times to Conduct Surveys

An important aspect of preparing for a walk-through survey is determining the most appropriate **time** for conducting it. This depends greatly on the type of work being investigated, when a particular work process is scheduled for operation, and environmental conditions within the workplace because each of these factors can affect the levels of exposure to a hazard. Timing should be such that accurate peak exposure times and levels can be determined.

Areas of Particular Concern

There are certain **areas of the workplace that are of particular concern** when conducting a worksite walk-through survey. These are places where the potential for exposure to hazardous conditions is high, and therefore should be monitored closely and investigated routinely so that the potential for illness or injury can be eliminated or reduced. Some examples of these types of working conditions are areas with extreme noise or heat, poor ventilation, awkward/harmful positioning, a potential for exposure to radiation, and areas with equipment and machinery operations.

Frequency of Surveys

The **frequency** of worksite walk-through surveys depends on two things: the type of work and changes in procedures. If the type of work or work process contains either many hazards or frequent exposure to just a few hazards, walk-through surveys should be conducted more frequently than instances where there are relatively few potential occupational health and safety hazards. Any time there is a change in work procedures, a worksite walk-through survey should be conducted to assess if there are new potential hazards. Regardless of the presence of potentially hazardous conditions, walk-through surveys should be conducted at some level on a regular basis. Ultimately, it is up to the occupational health professional to determine how frequently a survey should be conducted to maintain a safe and healthy environment.

Worksite Walk-Through Report

Once the survey is complete and all necessary data gathered and analyzed, a **report** must be generated. The purpose of this report is to present results and recommendations that will help to maintain a safe and healthy work environment. The report should contain information about data analysis, recommendations for the remediation of hazardous conditions, and a cost-benefit analysis associated with each recommendation. A copy of the report must be maintained in the occupational health offices, as well as distributed to relevant personnel and management. Along with the full report, a summary report should be provided to management highlighting the key points.

Improving Occupational Health and Safety Programs

The **end result of conducting a survey** is the enhancement and improvement of an occupational health and safety program. This is accomplished through assessing and improving hazard prevention and control strategies; using survey results to institute new programs, policies, and procedures, as well to justify the institution of safer equipment; and focusing on a system of quality control related to occupational health and safety issues.

Personal Protective Equipment

When designing control strategies to reduce or eliminate a hazardous condition, it is important to assess the most effect methods of control. As a whole, the use of **personal protective equipment** as a control strategy is considered the least effective of all potential control strategies. This is for two reasons. First of all, it does not remove the source of the hazard. Secondly, the equipment must be reliable and personnel in compliance with its use in order for it to be effective. If it is deemed appropriate to employ personal protective equipment as a control strategy, the equipment used must be appropriate to the hazard being remediate, it must be the proper size for those who are going to use it, all employees must be trained on correct use with a system for monitoring and enforcement in place, and the equipment must be regularly inspected and maintained.

Behavioral Safety Program

While OSHA does not mandate a specific **behavioral safety program**, it does recommend that one be in place. Behavioral safety programs vary, but tend to have similar elements:

- **Observations**: A consultant or trained employee conducts worksite observations to identify safe and unsafe behaviors as well as hazards (poor lighting, fatigue, inadequate PPE) that may lead to unsafe behaviors.
- **Checklists**: Observations are conducted using a checklist that includes ergonomics, housekeeping, PPE available and in use, and safe practices/driving. Each action and each condition in the checklist is checked as safe or unsafe.
- **Action plan**: An action plan to develop alternative safe behaviors is formulated after speaking with workers about the reasons for the unsafe behavior/conditions.
- **Positive reinforcement**: A system of rewards for utilizing safe behaviors is developed.
- **Evaluation**: Ongoing evaluation of progress is carried out, such as through reviewing incident reports and sick time as well as through further observations.

Standards and Regulations

Federal Regulations

Occupational Health Standards

Role of the EPA

The **Environmental Protection Agency** (EPA) works cooperatively with OSHA to support occupational health standards. In some cases, authority may overlap between the agencies, and they may carry out joint inspections. While OSHA focuses on the workplace itself, the EPA is charged with protecting public health and the environment (particularly focusing on air and water pollution), which affect the workplace, through various functions:

- Ensuring compliance with federal statutes/regulations.
- Setting clean water standards.
- Registering antimicrobial and disinfectant products
- Monitoring and controlling air pollution.
- Setting requirements for cleanup of toxic wastes.
- Levying fines for noncompliance.
- Setting standards and rules.
- Conducting technical reviews, such as audits and different studies.
- Conducting public hearings on health-related matters.
- Issuing permits and licenses.
- Carrying out compliance inspections.
- Providing guidance regarding mold and radon.
- Investigating violations.
- Evaluating research.
- Enacting laws to ensure environmental protection, such as Asbestos Hazard Emergency Response Act, Clean Air Act, Clean Water Act, Toxic Substances Control Act, and Safe Drinking Water Act.

Role of the FDA

The **Food and Drug Administration** (FDA) collaborates with OSHA and other agencies in the establishment of standards and compliance regulations that affect the workplace. The FDA has established current good manufacturing processes for food production and dietary supplement production (21 CFR 117) and requires hazard analysis and risk-based preventive measures. The FDA's role in occupational health standards includes:

- Regulating medical devices, such as respirators, to ensure that they are safe to use and that safety hazards are identified.
- Inspecting manufacturing facilities and conducting sampling and tests to ensure workers and the public protection from electronic product radiation.
- Inspecting facilities that produce food products and identifying safety concerns and violations.
- Evaluating results of manufacturer's tests and quality control programs.
- Ensuring that state standards meet minimum federal requirements.
- Ensuring safety of drugs, vaccines, and biological products.

- Regulating tobacco products.
- Identifying food safety violations.
- Protecting employees who report violations of food/drug handling/production or refuse to participate in work-required violations.

OSHA Standards for Respiratory Protection

OSHA has standards for **respiratory protection** (29 CFR 1910.134) that apply to general industry, shipyards, marine terminals, longshoring, and construction to protect workers who may be exposed to contaminated air from dusts, fogs, fumes mists, gases, smokes, sprays, or vapors:

- Respirators should be appropriate for the type and amount of contamination and may include air purifying respirators, atmosphere supplying respirators, demand respirators, dust masks, and escape-only respirators. Respirators must be NIOSH-certified and provided by the employer.
- Each employer must have in place a respiratory protection program that outlines procedures and requirements for respirator use. The respiratory protection programs should include procedures for selecting respirators, medical evaluation of employees required to use respirators, fit testing procedures, procedures for use, cleaning, disinfecting, repairing, inspecting and discarding respirators. Additionally, the program should include procedures to improve air quality, training (respiratory hazards, use of respirators, and when not to use respirators), and procedures for evaluating the program.

Confined Spaces

Confined spaces are those that are not intended for habitation or use by people but may be entered for work purposes. Typically, confined spaces may have limited/restricted entry and exit. Confined spaces include tanks, silos, storage bins, pits, manholes, tunnels, ductwork, pipes, and vessels. A permit-required confined space is one that may contain a hazardous environment, material that may engulf a person, walls that converge inward, tapering areas, sloping floors, unguarded machinery, or other hazardous materials. OSHA standards (29 CFR 1910, 1915, 1917, 1926) that apply include those for general industry, shipyard/maritime employment, and construction. It is critical to identify confined spaces, evaluate risks, and take preventive actions. Any confined space that poses a risk (deficient oxygen, atmospheric hazard/toxin) must be classified as permit-required and tested before and after entry and monitored continually while the person is in the space. The person must be provided the necessary safety equipment/PPE.

Clinical Nursing Guidelines

Independent Nursing Strategies

When **independent nursing strategies** are employed at the workplace, the nurse does not rely on a physician for direction. Instead, the nurse assesses the individual and comes up with the appropriate nursing interventions. This is very appropriate in a work setting where the occupational health nurse knows the work environment, collects data on occupational health illness and injury, and is trained in the necessary aspects of health and safety. However, because a nurse is not a physician, it is important that they know their limitations and seek out a physician referral when necessary. This means that the nurse must know what illnesses, injuries, signs, and symptoms require a physician's attention. If medical interventions are prescribed by a physician and delegated to the nurse, the nurse must be sure that these interventions are within both the technical capabilities and legal scope of nursing practice before executing them.

Effects of Standardized Care in Nursing

Standardized care in nursing helps to improve both the quality and consistency of care. It provides a nurse with the ability to assess a health problem and apply the most appropriate nursing interventions. The nurse assesses the signs and symptoms of a health issue and then applies a specific treatment option with very precise results in mind. This is a way to focus a program's approach to nursing so that a constant quality of care can be offered. Within standardized care, however, there needs to be room for the nurse to tailor the intervention to specific cases. In particular, the nurse must be well aware of red flags that alert them to complications or modifications to indicated interventions.

Clinical Nursing Guideline Development

Defining Parameters of Care and Management

Clinical nursing guidelines are used to help define parameters of care and management. They specify the actions that a nurse can legally take when performing their duties. Clinical nursing guidelines are particularly useful within the realm of occupational health and safety because the occupational health nurse is often the only trained medical professional in the program. In defining the limits of nursing practice, they also provide guidance as to specific nursing goals, maintaining a consistent quality of care, the need for record-keeping in maintaining quality assurance, and accountability within the nursing profession.

Development

Clinical nursing guidelines are necessary tools in delineating the limits of nursing care and administration. They specify the actions that a nurse can legally take when performing their duties. There are several steps to developing clinical nursing guidelines. The first step is to conduct a thorough review of current literature so that the most up-to-date methods and interventions are employed. Another essential element to the development of clinical nursing guidelines is the use of other medical professionals. They can provide valuable information on both current and new techniques in medicine. Finally, a review of occupational health records can give information on health trends within the workforce or other population groups. While it is important that any nursing guidelines provide the most accurate and up-to-date information for use in clinical settings, it is also imperative that they do not replace the critical thinking skills necessary in effective nursing.

Maintaining Guidelines

Once clinical nursing guidelines are developed, they must be **maintained**. This means that they must be regularly evaluated and updated by qualified medical personnel to keep them current, relevant, and in compliance with legal requirements. A review should be conducted at a minimum of once a year, with additional reviews conducted as seen fit. Updates to guidelines should always be dated and a current copy must be kept on file in both the occupational health unit, as well as any other relevant location throughout the workplace (such as departments where they are actively being used).

Emergency Response

Superficial Injuries

Abrasions and Lacerations

An **abrasion** is an injury where the surface of the skin is torn or rubbed off. A **laceration** is a cut or tear that can be either on the surface of the skin or go deeper to include the muscle. A piece of skin that is torn, but is still attached is called an **avulsion**. Abrasions and lacerations are usually caused by contact with hard, sharp pieces of equipment or from falls. The characteristics of an abrasion include pain, very little bleeding, and foreign objects many times imbedded in the injury. The characteristics of a laceration include a sharp, jagged edge to the injury, a great deal of bleeding with damage to tissue, nerves, and blood vessels possible. Both types of wounds carry with them a risk of infection and tetanus contamination.

A typical occupational health department's **policy and objectives** for treating an abrasion or laceration include the following: Assess the type and seriousness of the injury in the occupational health unit, verify tetanus immunization, control bleeding, and take steps to prevent infection.

Assessments and Interventions

The **clinical assessments and interventions** applied to treating an abrasion or laceration are as follows:

- Elevate injured body part and apply pressure to stop the bleeding.
- Clean the wound with a mild antiseptic solution and water.
- Use sterile-strips to close a laceration if necessary.
- Apply antibiotic ointment.
- Apply sterile dressing if needed (minor abrasions can be left uncovered).
- Verify tetanus immunization. If necessary, administer tetanus immunizations within 24 hours.
- Educate employee as to proper care of the wound (clean and dry dressing, change dressing regularly, clean wound regularly and assess for infection, limit activity to avoid worsening or re-injury).
- Educate employee on the signs and symptoms of infection (localized redness, warmth, tenderness, swelling, pain, or fever).

Referral Policy for Medical Action/Attention and Follow-Up Actions

The typical **referral policy** for medical action/attention and the **follow-up actions** necessary when treating an abrasion or laceration are as follows:

- **Referral:**
  - Any serious open wound or wound that cannot be effectively closed with sterile-strips.
  - Material embedded in the wound.
  - A cut with a loose flap of skin.
  - Any serious cut to the hands, fingers, feet, or toes, or over a joint.
  - Human or animal bite.
  - Laceration to the face.
  - Uncontrolled/excessive bleeding.
  - Contaminated wound.
  - Any signs of infection.
- **Follow-up:**
  - Assess wound for the presence of infection.
  - Evaluate worksite for potential hazards.
  - Make recommendations to reduce or eliminate the potential for future injuries.

Strains

A **strain** is an overstretching of a part of the musculature ("pulled muscle") that causes microscopic tears in the muscle or tendon, usually resulting from excess stress, overuse of the muscle, blunt trauma, or overstretching. Common sites for strains include the ankle, back, and hamstrings. Onset of pain is usually sudden with local tenderness on use of the muscle. Strains are classified according to severity:

- **1st degree:** This injury is relatively mild and symptoms, such as slight discomfort and tenderness to palpation, may be delayed until the following day.
- **2nd degree:** Pain is usually felt on injury with tenderness on palpation and decreased passive and active range of motion, depending upon the site of injury. There may be signs of injury, such as edema and bruising.
- **3rd degree:** The muscle or tendon is completely ruptured and pain occurs with injury. A defect may be palpable. Often there is extensive edema and bruising from injury to vasculature. Strength and loss of range of motion varies according to site of injury.

Occupational risk factors include heavy lifting, improper ergonomics, twisting. Treatment includes RICE (rest, ice, compress, elevate) and transport to ED if person hears or feels "popping, is unable to walk, edema and pain are significant, or the strain is associated with a laceration.

SPRAINS

A **sprain** is damage to a joint, with a partial rupture of the supporting ligaments, usually caused by wrenching or twisting that may occur with a fall. The rupture can damage blood vessels, resulting in edema, tenderness at the joint, and pain on movement with pain increasing over 2-3 hours after injury. An avulsion fracture (bone fragment pulled away by a ligament) may occur with strain, so x-rays rule out fractures. Sprains may be classified according to severity:

- **1st degree:** This is a relatively mild degree of injury, usually associated with good range of motion and mild pain. Swelling may vary considerably, depending upon whether vessels are disrupted by the sprain.
- **2nd degree:** This comprises a wide range of signs and symptoms, as there is further injury and partial rupture of the ligaments. Usually range of motion is limited by pain. Edema and bruising are usually present but vary in degree. The joint may be somewhat unstable.
- **3rd degree:** This involves total rupture of the ligament with immediate marked pain (although sometimes less than with 2nd degree), bruising, edema, and decreased range of motion. The joint is usually markedly unstable.

Occupational risk factors include strenuous activity, slippery (icy, wet) surfaces, uneven surfaces, use of ladders. Treatment includes RICE (rest, ice, compress, elevate) and transport to ED if unable to bear weight or use joint.

Amputation and Bleeding Injuries

Amputations

Amputation is defined as the severance of a body part. The characteristics of amputation include the exposure of bone, heavy bleeding, and shock. There are always potential complications associated with an amputation. These include infection, shock, and severe physical disability.

A typical occupational health department's **policy and objectives** for treating amputation include the following:

- Provide immediate emergency medical treatment within the occupational health unit.
- Take steps to recover and save the severed body part.

Assessments and Interventions

The **assessments and interventions** typically applied to treating amputation in an occupational health program are as follows:

- Assess openness of airway, give oxygen if necessary.
- Assess the extent of the wound and apply pressure to control bleeding.
- Support and immobilize injured body part.
- Irrigate the wound using sterile saline or tap water, cover with sterile pads.
- Provide immediate transportation to the hospital.
- Notify healthcare transporters if foreign objects are suspected in the wound.
- Never compromise the employee's health to save the severed body part.
- Clean severed part and wrap in sterile gauze, towel, or sheet.
- Cover the severed part with a wrap wet with sterile saline or lactated Ringer's solution.
- Never immerse the severed part in any solution.
- Seal severed part in container or bag, place bag in an ice-filled container.
- Maintain the anatomical position of the severed part.
- Record the time the amputation occurred.

Referral Policy for Medical Action/Attention and Follow-Up Actions

The typical **referral policy** for medical action/attention and the **follow-up actions** necessary when treating an amputation are as follows:

- **Referral** - Emergency medical treatment should be provided on site, but transportation to a hospital for evaluation and treatment should be arranged for as soon as possible. With correct care and treatment, the amputated part can often be saved and surgically reattached. It is important to note that one should never compromise the employee's life to save the amputated part.
- **Follow-up** - The employee should be educated on proper safety measures, rehabilitation, management of disability, and possible return to work. Because of the potential for disability, it is important to provide the employee with the necessary physical and psychological support.

Bleeding Injuries

OSHA standards require that some types of work include first aid training for all or some workers because of the risk of **bleeding** or other injuries, including logging employees, those working in remote substations (electric power), and commercial divers. Some industries, such as shipyards and construction work require that first aid supplies (gauze, tourniquets, compresses, and hemostatic dressings) be readily available because of the high incidence of bleeding injuries. While OSHA does not require that all worksites have on-site workers certified in first aid, it recommends this practice. Emergency response to bleeding injuries includes:

- Remove clothing and debris about the wound but do not probe the wound or take time to clean it.
- Apply compression (continual) with a sterile dressing or clean cloth to stop bleeding. A compression dressing may be applied (avoid pressure on the eye or on objects imbedded in the wound). If the dressing bleeds through, apply further dressings on top. If the wound is on an extremity, elevate the extremity.
- Position injured person reclining and maintain body heat.
- If available, a tourniquet may be applied or hemostatic dressing (such as QuickClot®) to control hemorrhage.
- Transport person to ED as soon as possible.

Burns

Thermal Burns

A **thermal burn** is defined as damage to tissue as a result of exposure to fire or a hot substance. Burns are classified into three different categories based on severity:

- A **first-degree burn** involves just the surface of the skin (epithelial layer) and is characterized by reddening of the skin (erythema) and pain.
- **Second-degree burns** include part of the dermal layer and are characterized by severe pain, erythema, blister formation, and cell fluid loss.
- **Third degree burns** are the most severe with damage occurring to the entire dermal layer of skin, as well as some muscle and bone. This type of burn is characterized by a black, white, or leathery appearance to the skin; excessive fluid loss; and shock.

Typical **policy and objectives** for treating a thermal burn include the following: Remove employee from heat or fire and assess the severity of damage. Stabilize the burn victim, treat minor burns immediately, and provide symptom relief for more severe burns. Immediate hospital transport is necessary for serious burns.

Assessments and Interventions

The **assessments and interventions** typically applied to treating a thermal burn include the following:

- Remove employee from the source of heat/flames and extinguish fire if possible.
- Check for unobstructed airway, apply oxygen if necessary.
- Assess extend and degree of burn.
- Examine employee for additional injuries, take vital signs.
- Cool burned area with tap water to no more than 20% of burned area for 10 minutes.
- If possible, remove clothing (do not disturb clothing that has adhered to the burned area).
- Cover burn with dry, clean, sterile dressing; never apply ice.
- Check for signs of smoke inhalation.
- Give intravenous Lactated Ringer's solution if necessary.
- Elevate burned areas.
- Never break blisters or apply ointments, creams, or topical anesthetics.
- Prevent shock.
- Transport to a hospital as necessary.

Referral Policy for Medical Action/Attention and Follow-Up Actions

The typical **referral policy** for medical action/attention and the **follow-up actions** necessary when treating a thermal burn are as follows:

- **Referral** - Immediate referral for medical attention should be sought in the following cases:
  - Burns that involve hands, face, eyes, feet, or perineum.
  - Electrical or inhalation burns.
  - Burns that also have other major traumas associated with them.
  - Any second-degree burn that covers more than 10% of the body.
  - Any third-degree burn.

- **Follow-up:**
    - Provide employees with information about signs and symptoms of infection.
    - Tell employees to keep the burned area elevated for at least 24 hours.
    - Change the dressing on the burn as needed.
    - Assess the burn area for infection.
    - Assess worksite for potential hazards and risks that can be eliminated.

SUNBURN

A **sunburn** is defined as exposure to ultraviolet (UV) light that results in damage/burning at the surface of the skin. It is characterized by the dilation of capillaries, redness and swelling (erythema), tenderness, edema, and sometimes the formation of blisters. It can also cause system-wide effects, such as headache, nausea, chills, fever, and sensitivity to light.

A typical occupational health department's **policy and objectives** for treating a sunburn include the following:

- Assess the burn and history of sun exposure in the occupational health unit.
- Provide necessary symptom relief.

ASSESSMENTS AND INTERVENTIONS

The **assessments and interventions** typically applied to treating a sunburn include the following:

- Obtain the following information: Length of most recent sun exposure, the use of sun protection, and the use of any photosensitive drugs.
- Assess the employee's skin and make note of any areas of redness, tenderness, blistering, abnormal moles, and lesions.
- Provide necessary symptom relief.
- If there is blistering with persistent pain, puncture any large blisters using a sterile needle, leaving the top skin of the blister intact.
- Recommend to employee the following home-administered symptom relief procedures: Cool baths, soothing lotions, and aloe vera. For more serious sunburns, recommend a lukewarm colloidal oatmeal bath for 20 minutes.

REFERRAL POLICY FOR MEDICAL ACTION/ATTENTION AND FOLLOW-UP ACTIONS

The typical **referral policy for medical action/attention** and the **follow-up actions** necessary when treating a sunburn are as follows:

- **Referral:**
    - Any signs and symptoms of infection.
    - A second-degree burn that covers more than 10% of the body.
    - Any third-degree burn.
- **Follow-up** - A follow-up consultation should include the following recommendations to reduce future UV exposure and skin damage:
    - Avoid exposure to the sun between 10AM and 3PM (when sun exposure is the greatest).
    - Do not use tanning booths, sun lamps, and tanning promoters.
    - Use sunscreen with a high protection factor that blocks both UVB and UVA rays.
    - Provide employee with information on the harmful effects of UV light (such as sunburn and skin cancers).

Cardiovascular and Neurological Injuries

Cardiovascular Emergencies and Use of AEDs

Workers may experience **cardiovascular emergencies**, such as cardiac arrest, while in the workplace, and prompt response may be critical to life-saving. Emergency defibrillation is done for acute ventricular fibrillation or ventricular tachycardia with no audible or palpable pulse; it is ineffective for asystole or pulseless electrical activity. Defibrillation delivers an electrical discharge through paddles applied to both sides of the chest. Automated external defibrillators (AEDs) are frequently available in the workplace. Procedure:

1. Immediately begin chest compressions at the rate of 100 - 120 per min while awaiting AED.
2. Turn on the AED.
3. Apply pads to chest (position may vary according to manufacturer). Infants and small children: If pads may touch, apply one to chest and one to back.
4. Plug in connector if necessary.
5. Do not touch patient while AED analyzes heart rhythm.
6. Follow directions for shocking and warn others to stand clear.
7. Continue CPR if no resuscitation beginning with compressions for 2 minutes between repeat defibrillations.

If the patient is wet, wipe off the chest before applying pads. Remove any transdermal patches on the chest, and shave excessive hair before applying pads. If the patient has an implanted device, the pads should be placed at least 1 inch (2.5 cm) away.

Contusions

A **contusion** is an injury to the soft tissue of the body where the skin is not broken. Contusions (commonly known as bruising) are most often caused by a direct hit or fall and are characterized by localized hemorrhaging (ecchymosis), pain swelling, and discoloration.

A typical occupational health department's **policy and objectives** for treating a contusion include the following:

- Assess the injury in the occupational health unit.
- Determine the severity and scope of the injury.
- Provide employee with symptom relief.

Assessments and Interventions

The **assessments and interventions** typically applied to treating a contusion include the following:

- Assess the contusion and surrounding area.
- Assess neurovascular status.
- Assess for peripheral nerve damage.
- Elevate injured part.
- Apply cold compress to area for ten minutes, and then 3-4 times thereafter to reduce swelling.
- Apply pressure bandages to reduce swelling.
- Apply warm moist heat to injured area after swelling is reduced.
- Administer analgesics as necessary.

REFERRAL POLICY FOR MEDICAL ACTION/ATTENTION AND FOLLOW-UP ACTIONS

The typical **referral policy for medical action/attention** and the **follow-up actions** necessary when treating a contusion are as follows:

- **Referral** - Most contusions can be adequately treated in the occupational health unit. A referral for medical action is necessary, however, if there are other more serious injuries associated with the contusion or if there is continued, persistent pain or disability.
- **Follow-up** - The employee should be provided with the following information:
  - Apply cold compresses or ice packs 3-4 times within the first 24 hours to reduce swelling.
  - Elevate and rest the injured part as much as possible.
  - Apply warm moist heat to the injured area after swelling is reduced (usually after 48 hours).
  - Report any persistent pain or disability to the occupational health unit.

WORK-RELATED HEAD INJURIES

CONCUSSIONS

Concussion is a brain injury in which structural damage is not apparent but neurological functioning is impaired. Patients may experience brief loss of consciousness after a head injury and may experience confusion and even bizarre behavior (if frontal lobe affected). Other symptoms include severe headache, somnolence, dizziness, lack of coordination, confusion, disorientation, inappropriate emotional response, nausea and vomiting. Symptoms are usually transient (lasting from minutes to hours), but up to 50% may have recurrent symptoms (such as difficulty concentrating, headaches, and dizziness) for months. American Academy of Neurology classification:

- **Grade 1:** Transient confusion without loss of consciousness with symptoms resolving in <15 minutes.
- **Grade 2:** Transient confusion without loss of consciousness with symptoms resolving in >15 minutes.
- **Grade 3:** Any loss of consciousness of any duration.

Emergency management includes supportive care and reassurance, monitoring vital signs and neurological status for signs of increasing intracranial pressure that may indicate more severe injury, and elevating head. Preventive measures include removing hazards from walkway, signage, handrails, proper use of footstools and ladders, and use of properly fitted protective helmet.

DIFFUSE AXONAL INJURY

Diffuse axonal injuries involve widespread brain damage, caused by traumatic shearing of neural axons from an impact injury, such as a motor vehicle accident, an assault, or a fall. Diffuse axonal injury is usually not evident on CT although multiple small focal hypo- or hyperdense lesions may be noted, and the patient is generally unconscious. Diffuse axonal injuries can result in a persistent unconscious state, coma, and chronic vegetative states:

- **Mild DAI**: Coma for up to 24 hours and may exhibit decorticate and decerebrate posturing.
- **Moderate DAI**: Longer period of coma with decorticate and decerebrate posturing.
- **Severe DAI**: Prolonged coma with episodes of hyperthermia, hypertension, and hyperhidrosis. Outcome is usually poor.

Emergency treatment includes supportive care, elevating head, and transport to ED for testing and further treatment. Patients who regain consciousness often need intensive rehabilitation. Preventive measures include PPE, environmental controls (safety ladders, safety belts), maintenance of motor vehicles, and adequate training.

Traumatic Brain Injury

Traumatic brain injury (TBI), sudden injury to the brain from an external force/impact, may have varying effects depending on the severity of the TBI. TBI may be primary with injury directly to the brain or secondary from injury to other parts of the body, (such as a traumatic injury to the chest). Occupational TBI may occur from falls, direct impact, secondary anoxia, assaults (including gunshot wounds) or acceleration/deceleration injuries (such as from a motor vehicle accident). Indications of a **mild TBI** may include headache, mild confusion, and disorientation; and a severe TBI, the inability to talk, walk, or carry out any ADLs with most patients located somewhere along the continuum. TBI may profoundly affect a person's cognitive abilities, physical abilities, and behavioral/emotional functioning. High risk occupations include construction, agriculture, fishing, and forestry. Emergency treatment includes supportive care, elevation of head, compression to control bleeding, and transport to ED for testing. Preventive measures include use of protective helmet (compliant with American National Standard for Industrial Head Protection) when work environment includes risk of falling object or exposed electrical conductors, appropriate safety equipment to prevent falls, including safety rails, appropriate maintenance of equipment/motor vehicles, following the hierarchy of controls, and adequate staff training.

Convulsions or Seizures

Convulsions (or seizures) are defined as the rapid and uncontrollable onset of muscular contractions and relaxations. They are characterized by the following: irregular contractions and relaxations of muscles, momentary loss of consciousness, and incontinence. Convulsions can be caused by epilepsy, meningitis, infections, heat cramps, brain lesions, eclampsia, diabetic hypoglycemia, and poisoning.

A typical occupational health department's **policy and objectives** for treating a convulsion or seizure include the following:

- Immediately assess employee in the occupational health unit and then refer for medical care.
- Take steps to keep the employee safe from injury during the seizure.

Assessments and Interventions

The **assessments and interventions** typically applied to treating a convulsion or seizure include the following:

- Keep employee resting/lying down.
- Assess for open airway after seizure.
- Maintain an open airway by lying employee down and moving head from side to side.
- Record information about the onset of the seizure including the time of onset, duration, origin of convulsion, type of contractions, presence of incontinence, head or other bodily injuries, and abnormal breath odor.
- Arrange for immediate medical care.

Referral Policy for Medical Action/Attention and Follow-Up Actions

The typical **referral policy for medical action/attention** and the **follow-up actions** necessary when treating a convulsion or seizure are as follows:

- **Referral** - After an employee is assessed in the occupational health unit, they must be referred for medical action.
- **Follow-up**
  - Occupational health department must work with employee's physician to establish a treatment and return to work plan.
  - The importance of taking prescribed medications as directed should be stressed.
  - Educate the employee about communication procedures for seizures.
  - Assess the compatibility of employee with previous job placement in light of seizure activity.

Eye Injuries

Flash Burn Eye Injuries

A **flash burn eye injury** is defined as an injury to the eye caused by exposure to extreme heat. In most flash burn eye injuries, both eyes are affected. This type of injury is characterized by pain, photophobia, inflammation, swelling, and tearing.

A typical occupational health department's **policy and objectives** for treating a flash burn eye injury include the following:

- Assess the injury in the occupational health unit, but arrange for immediate medical treatment.
- Provide employee with immediate symptom relief.

Assessments and Interventions

The **assessments and interventions** typically applied to treating a flash burn eye injury include the following:

- Assess the eye and surrounding tissue, as well as the employee's vision.
- Remove contact lenses immediately if found.
- Check eyes for the presence of foreign particles.
- Apply cold compresses for 5-minute periods until swelling is reduced.
- Give an analgesic as necessary.
- Refer for immediate medical attention.

Referral Policy for Medical Action/Attention and Follow-Up Actions

The typical **referral policy for medical action/attention** and the **follow-up actions** necessary when treating a flash burn eye injury are as follows:

- **Referral** - After an employee is assessed in the occupational health unit, they must be referred for immediate medical evaluation and treatment.
- Follow-up:
  - Assess the employee's vision.
  - Educate employee as to the use of proper eye protection.
  - Discuss the signs and symptoms of worsening of the injury.
  - Assess worksite to identify potential hazards and develop prevention strategies.

Fractures

Open Fractures

A **fracture** is defined as a break in a bone. In an **open fracture** (also called a compound fracture) there is an open wound associated with the area of the break. The characteristics of an open fracture include localized pain, deformity, unnatural position or movement, shortening of the affected limb, tenderness to touch, swelling, loss of range of motion, bone fragment protruding from wound, injured person assuming a protective posture. Some breaks can result in internal bleeding and shock.

A typical occupational health department's **policy and objectives** for treating an open fracture include the following:

- Assess the injury and determine severity.
- Stabilize the employee and injured limb.
- Arrange for immediate medical attention.

Assessments and Interventions

The **assessments and interventions** typically applied to treating an open fracture include the following:

- Maintain an open airway, breathing, and circulation.
- Control bleeding associated with open wound.
- Do not push any exposed bone back under the skin.
- Immobilize the injury with a splint.
- Treat for shock if necessary.
- Apply cold packs to reduce swelling.
- No not give anything to eat or drink.
- Do not elevate the injured limb if pelvic, spinal, or skull injuries are suspected.
- In the case of pelvic fracture, do not allow any movement.
- Arrange for immediate medical attention.

Referral Policy for Medical Action/Attention and Follow-Up Actions

The typical **referral policy for medical action/attention** and the **follow-up actions** necessary when treating an open fracture are as follows:

- **Referral** - If a fracture of any kind is suspected, the employee can be assessed and stabilized in the occupational health unit, however they must be referred for immediate medical evaluation and treatment.
- **Follow-up:**
  - Assess worksite to identify potential hazards and develop prevention strategies
  - Develop a return to work plan and assess the physical abilities of the employee before allowing them to return to work.

Closed Fractures

A **closed** (also called **simple**) **fracture** does not cause a break in the skin. The characteristics of a closed fracture include localized pain, deformity, unnatural position or movement, shortening of the affected limb, tenderness to touch, swelling, loss of range of motion, injured person assuming a protective posture. Some breaks can result in internal bleeding and shock.

A typical occupational health department's **policy and objectives** for treating a closed fracture include the following:

- Assess the injury and determine severity.
- Stabilize the employee and injured limb.
- Arrange for immediate medical attention.

Assessments and Interventions

The **assessments and interventions** typically applied to treating a closed fracture include the following:

- Maintain an open airway, breathing, and circulation.
- Assess for sensation, motion, swelling, and obvious deformity.
- Immobilize the injury with a splint.
- Treat for shock if necessary.
- Apply cold packs to reduce swelling.
- No not give anything to eat or drink.
- Unless it is otherwise recommended, elevate the limb after splinting.
- Do not elevate the injured limb if pelvic, spinal, or skull injuries are suspected.
- In the case of pelvic fracture, do not allow any movement.
- Arrange for immediate medical attention.

Referral Policy for Medical Action/Attention and Follow-Up Actions

The typical **referral policy for medical action/attention** and the **follow-up actions** necessary when treating an open fracture are as follows:

- **Referral** - If a fracture of any kind is suspected, the employee can be assessed and stabilized in the occupational health unit, however they must be referred for immediate medical evaluation and treatment.
- **Follow-up:**
    - Assess worksite to identify potential hazards and develop prevention strategies.
    - Develop a return to work plan and assess the physical abilities of the employee before allowing them to return to work.

Disease Management

Disease Process

Management of Disease Processes Resulting from Workplace Environment

Irritant/Contact Dermatitis

Irritant/Contact dermatitis is a localized response to contact with an allergen, resulting in a rash that may blister and itch. Common allergens include poison oak, poison ivy, latex, benzocaine, nickel, and preservatives, but there is a wide range of items preparations and products to which people may react. People may need work accommodations (PPE, change of environment) to reduce exposure to the allergen. Treatment includes:

- Identifying the causative agent through evaluating the area of the body affected, careful history, or skin patch testing to determine allergic responses.
- Corticosteroids to control inflammation and itching.
- Soothing oatmeal baths.
- Caladryl® lotion to relieve itching.
- Antihistamines to reduce allergic response.
- Lesions should be gently cleansed and observed for signs of secondary infection.
- Antibiotics are used only for secondary infections as indicated.
- Rash is usually left open to dry.
- Avoidance of allergen will prevent recurrence.

Occupational Asthma

Occupational asthma is triggered by something (fumes, gases, allergens) the worker encounters in the workplace and may occur immediately after contact or may develop over a period of weeks, months, or years. Up to 250 causative agents have been identified to date. Agents that are most commonly associated with occupational asthma include dust (grain, wood), pollens, tobacco, gums, synthetic dyes, isocyanates, inorganic chemicals, rosin, formaldehyde, and pharmaceuticals. A careful history and observation of symptoms is important in diagnosis, which may also include bronchial provocation and spirometric testing (both before and after work exposure). Once the triggering agent is identified, avoiding exposure is critical to controlling the symptoms although the symptoms may persist for years. Treatment usually includes bronchodilators to relieve wheezing and shortness of breath. Occupational exposure may occur in a wide range of occupations and workplaces, including bakeries, factories, coal mines, and hospitals. Preventive measures include compliance with health/safety regulations and guidelines, reducing exposure to allergens, use of PPE, establishment of surveillance program, training workers regarding potential hazards, and eliminating smoking.

Acute Respiratory Distress

Acute respiratory distress syndrome (ARDS) may result from exposure to smoke or toxic fumes in the workplace or severe injury that results in lung damage. Damage to the vascular endothelium and increase in the permeability of the alveolar-capillary membrane cause pulmonary edema as the alveoli fill with blood and protein-rich fluid and collapse. Atelectasis with hyperinflation and areas of normal tissue occur as the lungs "stiffen." Hypoxemia and tachypnea increase as the body tries to compensate to maintain a normal $paCO_2$. Symptoms occur within 72 (usually 24-48) hours of serious injury with marked dyspnea, productive cough (frothy white/pink sputum). Hypotension and tachycardia may occur. Emergency treatment includes removing patient from source of toxic exposure, oxygen therapy, and transport to ED. Endotracheal intubation and mechanical ventilation may be needed to maintain oxygen saturation above 90% if oxygen saturation falls. Untreated, the condition results in respiratory failure, multi-organ failure, and a mortality rate of 5-30%.

Controlling Diabetes at Work

Workers with diabetes must be allowed to manage their condition in the workplace. They need to maintain their routine schedule for meals and glucose testing to prevent complications and may need a private space for testing and injections. Accommodations for self-care may include the ability to monitor glucose levels (frequency may vary), space or refrigeration for storing supplies (glucose, insulin, syringes), ability to obtain food and drinks as needed, and adequate break time if the person has suffered a complication, such as an episode of hypoglycemia, needs to eat or drink, or needs to use the bathroom frequently. Some patients with peripheral neuropathy, ulcers, or amputations resulting from diabetes may require accommodations for decreased mobility or asked to be reassigned to different work. Others may require accommodations, such as screen readers, larger computer monitors, and magnifying aids for visual impairment. For diabetes, type 2, diabetic workers may wish others to be informed and educated about the signs of hyperglycemia and hypoglycemia and appropriate emergency response. In some cases, workers may need time off to adjust medication schedule or to treat complications.

Risk Factors in Workers with High Cholesterol and/or Hypertension

High cholesterol increases the risk of workers developing **hypertension,** and both increase the risk that the worker will develop stroke, coronary artery heart disease, kidney disease, and/or heart attack. Those with hypertension should avoid:

- Shift work: Can lead to or exacerbate hypertension.
- Working with time constraints: Increases stress.
- Working long hours without adequate rest: Increases hypertension.
- Stressful working conditions: Increases hypertension, can lead to an increase in the level of LDL, which in turn increases health risks.
- Work that requires excessive physical exertion or strain: Increases hypertension.
- Cold work environment: Vasoconstriction leads to hypertension.
- Work in hot/humid area: May result in increased stress and postural hypotension.

Workers should especially be aware of poor eating habits (snacks, fast foods high in fat and sodium) often associated with the workplace as these can lead to increased weight, cholesterol levels, and hypertension. Workers should try to find ways to alleviate stress, exercise, and eat healthy meals, and some may require medications to reduce cholesterol level and hypertension.

Wound Care for Preexisting Wounds

If a worker has an **existing wound**, then the worker should be cleared for work by a physician to ensure the safety of the worker and others in the workplace. Those with existing wounds are especially at risk of acquiring infections, such as *Staphylococcus* and MRSA, if they work in the healthcare field, veterinary services, correctional facilities, gyms, or daycares, or if they work with livestock. Workers with existing wounds should try to avoid crowding, touching contaminated surfaces, and close contact with others and should practice frequent handwashing as well as disinfecting their workspace. Workers generally don't need to be excluded from work unless their wounds produce copious amounts of purulent discharge that cannot be contained with appropriate dressings. Existing wounds should be kept covered with dressings. In some cases, work accommodations may be needed. If dressings must be changed at work, soiled dressings should be double-bagged and disposed of properly.

Chronic Pain Management for Workers

Chronic pain management is a concern for many workers, especially as the workforce ages so pain management is a concern for the occupational health nurse. Chronic pain may be related to a disease process, such as arthritis or peripheral neuropathy, or to work injuries, such as low back pain, which is common in industries that involve heavy lifting or bending. Interventions may include:

- **Pharmacologic:** Acetaminophen and ibuprofen are the mainstays of nonprescription pain management. Some workers with severe pain may resort to the use of opioids, but they tend to be ineffective for chronic pain and increase risk of addiction. Some workers may benefit from topical use of diclofenac or capsaicin while others from oral anticonvulsants (such as gabapentin) or TCAs.
- **Non-pharmacologic**: Workers should be encouraged to maintain a healthy diet, get adequate sleep, and exercise to tolerance. Complementary therapies to help reduce or control chronic pain may include_relaxation, visualization, acupuncture, music therapy, aromatherapy, Ayurveda, biofeedback, chiropractic medicine, hypnosis, meditation, massage, traditional Chinese medicine, yoga, naturopathy, acupuncture, and Tai Chi.

Case Management

Aspects of Case Management

Coordination and Service Delivery

Coordination and service delivery is one of the five knowledge domains essential to occupational health case management. The following information and tasks fall under this knowledge domain:

- Understanding of the rules for the confidentiality of personal and medical information.
- Knowledge and understanding of medical terminology.
- Ability to take a complete and accurate health history.
- Ability to establish treatment goals and plans, as well as accurately communicate this information to the employee and necessary personnel.
- Knowledge and understanding of the medical referral process.

Physical and Psychological Factors

Physical and psychological factors are one of the five knowledge domains essential to occupational health case management. The following information and tasks fall under this knowledge domain:

- Ability to identify cases appropriate for management.
- Ability to assess the patient's health and safety needs, as well as be an advocate for the patient so that those needs are met.
- Knowledge and understanding of the physical and psychological characteristics associate with both illness and wellness.
- Ability to assist employees in establishing both short-term and long-term goals for a healthy life.

Benefit Systems and Cost-Benefit Analysis

Benefit systems and cost-benefit analysis is one of the five knowledge domains essential to occupational health case management. The following information and tasks fall under this knowledge domain:

- Ability to assess the quality and cost effectiveness of medical services.
- Knowledge and understanding of the steps in the of prior approval process.
- Ability to identify cases that should be referred for a different plan of care.
- Ability to research and determine the cost of any particular treatment plan.
- Knowledge and understanding of healthcare delivery systems and home health resources available to the patient.

Case Management Concepts

Case management concepts are one of the five knowledge domains essential to occupational health case management. The following information and tasks fall under this knowledge domain:

- Knowledge and understanding of the role that the case manager plays in an occupational health program, including case management philosophy, principles, and problem solving techniques.
- Ability to completely and accurately document case management services, as well as to assess the effectiveness of those services.

- Ability to apply planning and goal development techniques to the case management process.
- Knowledge and understanding of the legal issues associated with the case management process.

Community Resources

Community resources are one of the five knowledge domains essential to occupational health case management. The following information and tasks fall under this knowledge domain:

- Ability to effectively communicate the community resources available to employees (including the limitations of these resources).
- Knowledge and understanding of the different means available to assist employees with disabilities.
- Knowledge and understanding of the legal rights of those with disabilities (Americans with Disabilities Act.)
- Ability to effectively establish an employee support system that includes vocational counseling.

Influences on Employer-Related Costs of Healthcare Programs

There has been an increase in occupational health and disability case management programs in recent years, and with this comes an increase in the **costs** and **spending** associated with these programs. There are several factors that influence the employer-related costs of healthcare programs. These include (but are not limited to) any paid employee leave (sick, disability, workers' compensation), the cost of hiring and training workers to replace those on leave, the costs associated with healthcare benefits and insurance premiums, and an overall reduction in workplace productivity due to accident or illness.

Purposes of Occupational Health Case Management Program

The overall **goal of an occupational health case management program** is to meet the health and safety needs of the workforce in an efficient and cost-effective manner. The **four main purposes** of such a program are as follows:

1. Identify cases that would benefit from case management services.
2. Provide employees with healthcare services that are of the highest quality, while at the same time being cost-effective and efficient.
3. Ensure a healthcare system that is well organized so as to facilitate a speedy recovery.
4. Provide employees with the means and support necessary to return to work after an illness or injury.

Stages of Case Management Process

There are **six stages** that make up the **case management process**. The execution of each of the six stages in the correct and consecutive order is an important part of a well-organized and effective occupational health case management program. Without these stages, case management and healthcare services delivery become disorganized which can slow or prevent the full recovery of the patient. The six stages (in order) are as follows:

1. Case selection.
2. Assessment/problem identification.
3. Development and coordination of the case plan.
4. Implementation of the case plan.
5. Evaluation and follow-up.
6. Continuous monitoring, reassessing, and re-evaluating.

Case Selection

Case selection is the first stage of the case management process. In this stage, the patient is assessed and recommended for case management services. Early intervention is often the key to an effective case management program, allowing for the provision of necessary quality, efficient and cost-effective healthcare services. This is particularly the case with individuals that have chronic diseases (i.e. diabetes), high-risk conditions (i.e. AIDS), or work-related conditions that have the potential to develop high-risk injury or illness. During the case selection process, workers' compensation, group health, and disability claims can be analyzed to help identify high cost/high volume cases.

Assessment/Problem Identification

Assessment/problem identification is the second stage of the case management process. It occurs after it has been determined that an employee needs case management services. This stage involves the gathering of data to determine the employee's needs (including physical, social, financial, and psychological). Both personal and medical information go into the problem identification stage. This information can come from the employee, employer, the employee's family, the employee's primary physician, or health records. A Health Status Survey (filled out by the employee) is a simple yet effective means of information gathering necessary health and personal information.

General Assessment Data

The **general assessment data** that should be collected as a part of the assessment/problem identification stage of the case management process includes a health history and demographic information, medical status including any medications, nutritional status as it relates to employee health, financial status as it relates to ability to pay healthcare costs, ability to function in daily life, psychosocial status, cultural/religious background (in particular, those traditions that may impact health status or treatment options), community resources available to the employee, responsibilities of the employee to the company, and the responsibilities of the employer to meet the healthcare needs of the employee.

Development and Coordination of Case Plan

Development and coordination of a case plan is the third stage of the case management process. It entails developing an efficient and cost-effective plan of care for the patient. This stage of the case management process requires the cooperation of each of the individuals involved in the case including the patient, physician, family, payer, and specialists. In order to develop a plan of care that fits the needs of the patient, it is critical that the occupational health case manager have an accurate and thorough understanding of the situation, particularly any potential problems or complications that may arise. Goals and objectives are established for the plan of care so that the case manager has a way to determine its effectiveness. If the plan is determined to be ineffective or if the needs of the patient change, the case manager updates and changes the plan as necessary.

Implementation

Implementation is the fourth stage of the case management process. In this stage, the plan of care is implemented. If medical referral is necessary, it is the responsibility of the occupational health case manager to indicate the appropriate specialist. It is important to understand that the case manager is not responsible for actual treatment of the patient. They do, however, help coordinate the effort by monitoring the quality of care, providing necessary information to the patient (i.e. treatment options, community resources, benefits coverage), make arrangements for necessary home health equipment, instituting return to work policies including establishing necessary rehabilitation programs.

Evaluation and Follow-Up

Evaluation and follow-up is the fifth stage of the case management process. In this stage, the plan of care is evaluated and determined if it has been effective in reaching the established goals and objectives. This is a critical step in the case management process. The overall purpose of case management is to provide the oversight necessary if one is to provide quality healthcare that is also efficient and cost-effective. Thus, the evaluation stage plays a major role in preventing complications as well as reducing unnecessary or ineffective treatment options. Because assessing patient satisfaction is a part of the evaluation process, this stage allows employees to provide comments or concerns regarding the plan of care.

Continuous Monitoring, Reassessing, and Re-Evaluating

Continuous monitoring, reassessing, and re-evaluating is the sixth and final stage of the case management process. This is an on-going stage that does not end until the established goals and objectives are met and the case has been closed. As a part of this continuous monitoring step, the patient's health status, physical and emotional capabilities, as well as satisfaction with the program should assessed as a way to check if the plan of care is accomplishing what was established in the goals and objectives. If monitoring and evaluation indicate that the plan is not fulfilling its purpose, it is up to the occupational health case manager to modify it accordingly. The ultimate goal is an effective recovery and smooth return to work.

Indicators for Case Management Intervention

There are a number of **indicators that an individual's case should be recommended for management**. Some of these include (but are not limited to) the following:

- Ongoing symptoms/medication, including repeat surgeries or hospitalizations.
- Age of the employee, particularly if close to retirement.
- Work-related issues including problems with supervisor/coworkers or history of poor work performance.
- Complicated case including multiple diagnoses, a severe diagnosis, noncompliant with treatment, several healthcare providers, or many changes in healthcare providers.
- Workman's comp issues including a history of prior claims, fraudulent claims, or attorney involvement.
- Financial issues, including hardship or the potential for financial gain.
- Personal issues including unsatisfactory living conditions or the lack of a social/family support system.
- Admission to an extended care or transitional care facility.

Clinical Practice

Direct Clinical Care

Direct Care Services

There are a number of **direct care services** that may be available to employees through an occupational health program. These include (but are not limited to) clinical care geared towards treating both occupational and no occupational health issues, first aid and emergency care services, prenatal care, prevention and education services, health surveillance and monitoring, physical therapy, counseling services, and case management. Just which services are available depends on the company's priorities, the availability of community and emergency care, as well as the overall health of the workforce and hazard profile of the workplace.

Influences on Direct Clinical Care

There are a number of factors that **influence the direct clinical care** that is provided in a work setting. A company's attitude towards the types of services considered important plays the biggest role in the overall direct clinical care services offered. The need within the workforce also impacts these services. For example, if the work environment contains many potential hazards or if the overall workforce has numerous health issues (work or non-work related), there is a greater need for more services at the workplace. Likewise, if the workplace is too far from a hospital, if there are no community healthcare services available to the workers, or if there is a lack of health services benefit coverage, then the need for direct clinical services increases.

Benefits of Direct On-Site Clinical Services

As long as the services are high quality and cost-effective, there are a number of **benefits** that come with providing on-site clinical services at work. These include (but are not limited to) a decrease in absenteeism due to illness or injury, a decrease in company-absorbed costs due to absenteeism, opportunities to educate the workforce on health improvement and injury reduction, the chance to assess and monitor the health of the workforce and provide direct care services that meet these health needs. Just which services are available depends on the company's priorities, the availability of community and emergency care, as well as the overall health of the workforce and hazard profile of the workplace.

Absenteeism Program

An **absenteeism program** is designed to assess the reasons for absenteeism (missing work for planned or unplanned reasons) and to establish measures to reduce absenteeism. Absenteeism represents a major expense for employers (about $226 billion annually) and may include sick time, vacation time, absence because of work-related injury/illness or personal issues, or dysfunctional work environment. Absenteeism can negatively affect those who must do the work of those who are absent. Absenteeism and tardiness should be tracked to determine if patterns arise (particular individuals, days, or events). An absenteeism program should include:

- **Attendance policy:** Expectations regarding attendance and being on time should be outlined as well as the organization's definition of excessive absenteeism and tardiness and any disciplinary actions that may occur as a result.
- **Performance review**: Attendance should be considered as part of performance and workers should receive positive reinforcement for good attendance and adhering to the attendance policy.
- **Wellness program**: Focusing on improving health habits through smoking cessation, substance abuse treatment, emotional support, exercise, and diet.
- **Flexible work schedule**: Allowing workers to work from home or to have flexible work hours may reduce absenteeism.

Workplace Assessments

Types of Workplace Assessments

While a health assessment, monitoring, and surveillance program can incorporate many different health professionals (nurse, doctor, safety officer), it is often the occupational health nurse that is responsible for its implementation and management. Thus, it is important to understand the **different types of formal workplace assessments** that are a part of a health assessment, monitoring, and surveillance program. They are as follows:

- Preplacement Assessment
- Return to Work Assessment
- Job Transfer Assessment
- Periodic Health Monitoring
- Health Surveillance

Information for Accurate Health Assessment

A certain amount of information that is included in a workplace health assessment comes from the **employer**. This typically consists of the most up to date information about the worker's job. This includes information such as a complete job description and a job safety analysis. A **job safety analysis** includes a definition of the job and a description of the activities that make up the job. A JSA provides necessary information about the hazardous nature of the job such as its repetitiveness, any known potential hazards associated with the execution of the job, as well as relevant suggestions for the remediation of known hazardous conditions.

Preplacement Assessment

Workplace assessments are conducted to ensure the compatibility of the worker and job, thus minimizing the potential for worker injury or illness due to improper job placement. There are five different common types of workplace assessments. The preplacement assessment is one of them. It is conducted at the time of employment and is designed to assess and identify the most suitable job placement for the new employee, as well as for the purpose of gathering baseline data that the occupational health and safety nurse can use in future health assessment and monitoring activities. Without the preplacement assessment, it would be difficult to determine whether or not injuries or illnesses are as a result of work-or non-work-related exposures or stresses.

Objective and Subjective Data

There are five types of workplace assessments: preplacement assessment, return to work assessment, job transfer assessment, periodic health monitoring, and health surveillance.

A **preplacement assessment** is conducted at the time of employment and is designed to assess and identify the most suitable job placement for the new employee, as well as for the purpose of gathering baseline data that the occupational health and safety nurse can use in future health assessment and monitoring activities. Both **objective and subjective data** are incorporated into a preplacement assessment:

- Subjective data is personal in nature and can come from the worker, employer, or occupational health nurse. It includes information such as the personal and family health history of the worker, an occupational health history, and a review of the general health of the worker.
- Objective data is more of an actual measurement. It includes laboratory results, clinical measurements or tests, and the results of a physical examination conducted by a healthcare professional familiar with occupational health assessments.

Occupational Health History

As a part of the subjective data that is incorporated into a preplacement assessment, an **occupational health history** is taken. The basic components are as follows:

- Description of all jobs that the worker has ever participated in.
- Assessment of negative health effects due to exposures to potential hazards.
- Information about any signs and symptoms that could be indicative of occupational illness or injury.
- Information about lifestyle choices with known negative health effects such as smoking and drinking habits.

Physical Exam

As a part of the objective data that is incorporated into a preplacement assessment, workers are given a **physical examination**. This should be performed by a qualified health professional that is familiar with the occupational health and safety issues that face the worker in a given industry. The scope of the exam depends largely on the type of job that the worker is expected to perform and the hazards associated with it, with those systems that will be affected considered a priority. A preplacement physical exam provides valuable information so that recommendations can be made for the appropriate job placement of a new employee. It is also a way for the occupational health and safety nurse to gather baseline data that can be used in future health assessment and monitoring activities.

Laboratory and Clinical Measurement

As a part of the objective data that is incorporated into a preplacement assessment, a **series of laboratory and clinical measurements** are taken. Which tests are performed depends largely on the type of job that the worker is expected to perform and the hazards associated with it, with tests that focus on those systems that will be affected considered a priority. These tests serve several purposes: to collect baseline data for future exams/tests, as a part of mandated regulations, and to screen for negative health effects. Some of the tests that are usually a part of preplacement lab work include a complete blood count, urinalysis, and blood chemistry. The laboratory and clinical measurements taken during the preplacement process provide valuable information so that recommendations can be made for the appropriate job placement of a new employee. They are also a way for the occupational health and safety nurse to gather baseline data that can be used in future health assessment and monitoring activities.

Results and Job Compatibility

When making a recommendation for placement, the occupational health nurse can recommend that certain restrictions/reasonable modifications be completed before the worker begins the job. It is then up to the employer to attempt to meet the worker's needs for a safe and healthy work environment, or place them in a different job without those demands.

Refusal of Job Placement

Once a preplacement assessment is completed, it is up to a qualified health professional to determine the compatibility of the worker with the job. It is sometimes the case that a person is **refused placement** in a job based on the results of a preplacement assessment. In these cases, an individual can only be denied placement if they are not able to do the job safely. They CANNOT be denied a job if the assessment brings to light health condition that will increase insurance costs or if they are disabled but can do the job with reasonable accommodations.

Confidentiality Policies and Personal Health Information

Any personal health information that is accumulated during a preplacement assessment is strictly **confidential** and it is important that this information remain that way. It is the responsibility of the occupational health and safety nurse is to provide an employer with a recommendation as to an employee's ability to perform a job in a safe and healthy manner. Providing any personal health information to the employer with that recommendation is neither necessary nor allowed.

Return-to-Work Strategies

Rapid, Safe Return to Work

The **institution of a rapid, safe return to work policy** allows for an employee to return to work either part-time or to a modified duty job with the intention of promoting worker health, confidence, and productivity. It is often the case that the sooner an employee returns to work after an illness or injury, the quicker their recovery will be.

Return to Work Assessment

There are five different common types of workplace assessments. The **return to work assessment** is one of them. It is conducted after an employee has a long absence from work due to a work- or non-work-related illness or injury. The purpose of this assessment is to determine if the worker is capable of returning to their original job. In some cases, an illness or injury makes it impossible for the worker to return to their original job. In these instances, the occupational health nurse can recommend that certain restrictions/reasonable modifications be completed before the worker begins the job. It is then up to the employer to attempt to meet the worker's needs for a safe and healthy work environment, or place them in a different job without those demands.

Work Hardening

A **return to work assessment** is conducted when illness or injury has prohibited a worker from performing his/her job for an extended period of time. The principle reason for this type of assessment is to assess if the worker is physically and mentally able to return to their job after a long absence. If it is determined that the employee is not yet capable of returning to their original job without some form of physical conditioning, a "work hardening program" may be suggested. This a physical conditioning program where the worker completes a series of work-related tasks or activities that are progressively more physically demanding. The overall goal of a work hardening program is to slowly improve the worker's strength and resilience until they are fully recovered and able to return to their original job.

Modified/Transitional Duty and Complications with Serious Occupational Injuries

A return to work assessment is conducted when illness or injury has prohibited a worker from performing his/her job for an extended period of time. The principle reason for this type of assessment is to assess if the worker is physically and mentally able to return to their job after a long absence. If it is determined that the employee is not yet capable of returning to their original job, but is still able to work in some capacity, a recommendation for "**modified/transitional duty**" can be made. This allows the worker to continue working until they are fully recovered and able to return to their original job. A modified/transitional duty job is usually a modified version of the worker's previous job that is more in keeping with the individual's new needs and capabilities. If the worker never fully recovers from the illness/injury, the new modified job may become a permanent placement.

If the illness or injury is serious or chronic, the physical and psychological impacts may further delay and complicate the employee's return to work. In these cases, it may be necessary to refer the worker for additional services such as case management, rehabilitation, specialists, or counseling.

Job Transfer Assessment

Workplace assessments are conducted to ensure the compatibility of the worker and job, thus minimizing the potential for worker injury or illness due to improper job placement. There are five different common types of workplace assessments, and the **job transfer assessment** is one of them. It is conducted when a worker is expected to perform a different job from the one in which they were originally assessed and placed. In conducting this type of assessment, the occupational health professional compares the results of previous worker assessments to the new job's requirements and makes recommendations for job placement that reflect a safe and productive working environment.

Periodic Health Assessments

There are five different common types of workplace assessments, and the **periodic health assessment** is one of them. This type of assessment is conducted sporadically throughout an individual's employment to ascertain if the worker is still compatible with the job, to determine if there are any negative health effects related to the job, and to address and eliminate potential negative health effects before they develop into serious health problems.

Screening

Screening is one part of a periodic health assessment program. Screening is a method of identifying illness or injury before the onset of the signs and symptoms that would prompt an individual to seek medical attention. It consists of various examinations, tests, and procedures that are given to workers that are considered high risk for developing particular illnesses or diseases. While these tests are not necessarily diagnostic, they do, indicate when further testing is necessary, and thus contribute greatly towards the preventative side of an occupational health and safety program.

Biological Monitoring

Biological monitoring is the last part of a periodic health assessment program. Biological monitoring consists of the testing and detection of specific hazards and/or their by-products in the body fluids, exhaled air, and tissues of workers. It is important to note that biological monitoring only indicates the presence of a substance. It does not provide information about toxicity or negative health effects. Additional testing is necessary to gather this type of information.

Health Surveillance

Health surveillance is the final type of workplace assessment. Periodic health assessments are conducted sporadically throughout an individual's employment to ascertain if the worker is still compatible with the job, to determine if there are any negative health effects related to the job, and to address and eliminate potential negative health effects before they develop into serious health problems. Surveillance consists of the analysis of health information to identify particular procedures or problems in the workplace that could result in illness or injury. Surveillance activities can be directed at individuals, a department, a group of workers, or a specific occurrence in the workplace. They are an important aspect of the preventative side of an occupational health and safety program.

Health Education/Promotion

Counseling/Health Promotion

Role of Occupational Health Nurse as Employee Counselor

Some of the issues that an occupational health nurse may provide **counseling** for are as follows: Nutrition, exercise, substance abuse, marriage and divorce, birth and death, parenting issues, stress-related illness, psychological disorders such as anxiety and depression, as well as other major health-related events such as cancer and HIV/AIDS. When acting in the role of counselor, it is important that the occupational health nurse is skilled in all areas necessary to make accurate assessments and recommendations for appropriate care and referral services. At all times, an occupational health nurse must be acting within the legal limits of state nurse practice acts.

Counseling Points

There are many possible **counseling points** in which an occupational health nurse could provide counseling services. There are any number of physical, emotional, and psychological issues within the lives of the workers that may require counseling. For this reason, it is important that occupational health staff are educated and trained in a wide variety of areas. Within the realm of counseling, it is particularly necessary to take a multidisciplinary approach due to the many different counseling possibilities. When acting in the role of counselor, however, it is important that an occupational health nurse not be confused with a therapist. Thus, it is important that the occupational health nurse is skilled in all areas necessary to make accurate assessments and recommendations for appropriate care and referral services.

Occupational Stress as a Potential Counseling Opportunity

Stress is very common in the workplace. In fact, many workers believe that there is more on-the-job stress today than ten years ago. Therefore, if an occupational health nurse is to be involved in **occupational stress-related counseling,** it is important that they have an understanding of how it is defined and some of the factors that can lead to job stress. National Institute for Occupational Safety and Health (NIOSH, 1999) defines occupational stress as the harmful physical and emotional reactions that occur when the requirements of a job are not a fit for the worker. It can be a deficit in capabilities, resources, or needs of the worker. In any case, job stress ultimately results in poor health or injury. Some of the job conditions (as outlined by NIOSH, 1999) that can lead to job stress are poor task design, ineffective management styles, poor job-related interpersonal relationships, conflicting work roles, career concerns, and disagreeable environmental conditions.

Healthy People Program

Healthy People is a program that was first developed by the US Department of Health and Human Services in 1979. It is designed to deal with the preventable causes of disease, disability, and premature death with the goals of increasing the quality of life, increasing the length of life, and eliminating gaps and inequality in the healthcare system. It is divided into 28 focus areas, with each focus having specific goals. There are a total of 467 objectives designed to meet these goals. The current iteration of the program, **Healthy People 2020**, has a targeted timeframe for reaching the goals in 2020 (hence the name). The overarching emphasis of the Healthy People program is health education, promotion, and protection.

Leading Health Indicators

Leading Health Indicators are the key health problems in the country at present and are designed to assist in the development of health education, promotion, and protection activities. They provide information about the issues that have the potential to effect important health issues (such as behaviors, physical and social factors, and well as health system issues). They are based on the approximately 1200 goals and objectives outlined in "Healthy People 2020" and are intended to be used as building blocks for community health programs with the goals of increasing the quality of life, increasing the length of life, and eliminating gaps and inequality in the healthcare system.

Lifetime Health Monitoring Program

A **lifetime health monitoring program** consists of a regular (usually yearly) physical exam and laboratory tests to assess and monitor an individual's health through their lifetime. It is a preventative measure, intended to catch risk factors and recommend changes before they develop into disease, as well as to catch illness and disease while still treatable. Lifetime health monitoring programs were recommended by the American Medical Association in 1922, and have been the common practice for years. Recently, it has been determined that the same exams and tests every year for every person regardless of risk, is a waste of time and resources. In 1983 the American Medical Association endorsed a change to this type of health monitoring program, indicating that it was not necessary to perform a routine physical exam for everyone. Instead, each person should undergo an assessment of risk, and then the relevant procedures can be conducted relative to each person's individual needs.

Health Promotion and Health Protection

Health promotion and **health protection** both focus on the choices one makes to maintain a healthy lifestyle. There is a difference, however, between the approach that each takes and the motivating factors used to achieve this healthy lifestyle. The differences are illuminated in the following definitions:

- **Health promotion** – Behaviors and lifestyle choices that are motivated by the desire to actively live a healthy life and improve one's well-being.
- **Health protection** – Behaviors and lifestyle choices motivated by the desire to avoid sickness. This includes the early detection of disease and, once a disease has been detected, taking steps to maintain one's functional ability as allowed by the constraints of the disease.

Primary Prevention Activities

There are **three different levels of prevention**: primary, secondary, and tertiary.

Primary prevention, the first of three levels of prevention, focuses on eliminating or reducing the risk of disease by taking specific steps/actions that have this goal. Primary prevention activities fall into two categories, health promotion and risk reduction/prevention. Some examples of each are as follows:

- **Health Promotion**: Nutrition enhancement, exercise and fitness, reproductive health, health motivation enhancement.
- **Risk Reduction/Prevention**: Immunization, stress management, smoking cessation, risk factor appraisal, seat belt use, worksite walk-throughs, personal protective equipment use.

Secondary Prevention Activities

Secondary prevention, the second of three levels of prevention, deals with early detection of disease and taking steps to stop its progress. Implementing tests and physical examinations relative to risk group is an important aspect of this level of prevention. The key to effective secondary prevention is diagnosis and intervention while a disease is still treatable. Some examples of secondary prevention activities are as follows: Preplacement exams, periodic exams, health surveillance activities, screening programs, monitoring health/illness trend data, and nutrition education as it relates to disease control.

Tertiary Prevention Activities

Tertiary prevention, the third of three levels of prevention, is used when a disease is detected and stabilized, but irreversible. It focuses on maintaining the health of the individual and providing rehabilitation so that they can obtain the optimal level of health and well-being within the confines of the disease. With many diseases, although the condition is irreversible, a person can return to a normal life as long as lifestyle adjustments are made to manage the disease. The degree to which an individual can return to a normal, healthy life greatly depends on the disease and its progression. Some examples of tertiary prevention activities include disability management, case management, early return to work, chronic illness monitoring, chronic illness education, and substance abuse rehabilitation.

Health Promotion Programs

Health promotion programs are focused on improving health and quality of life. The ultimate goal of any health promotion program is to provide employees with the knowledge and understanding necessary to live a healthy life (both physically and emotionally). Some of the activities that are a part of this type of programming include physical fitness and weight management, stress reduction and management, smoking cessation, healthy eating habits, optimal self-care, substance abuse assistance, and life/work balance. Each of these activities has the dual purpose of promoting healthy lifestyle choices, while at the same time eliminating or reducing a risk factor for disease development.

Types

There are **three types of health promotion programs** that can help achieve the goals of improving health and quality of life. They are awareness, lifestyle change, and support environment programs:

- **Awareness programs** focus on providing information as a means of changing health attitudes and beliefs. They are geared towards individuals who need a better understanding of health and risk factors for developing disease.
- **Lifestyle change** programs go a step beyond awareness programs by using education and behavior modification techniques to assist individuals in making lifestyle changes that improve their overall health.
- **Supportive environment programs** promote healthy lifestyle choices by establishing and promoting an environment that encourages these types of behaviors. Friends, family, organizational cultures, coworkers, communities, and regulations all play a part in establishing this type of environment. Supportive environment programs tend to have the most lasting effects on the participants.

Health Promotion Program Model Phases

The **Health Promotion Program Model** is a framework that is useful in developing a health promotion program.

Assessment

Assessment is the first of four phases that makes up this model. During the assessment phase, the workplace is analyzed for its need of health promotion activities. This includes getting a better understanding of the level of corporate commitment to a health promotion program, the health education needs of the population being addressed, and the kinds of resources that are available for instituting health promotion activities. Each of these is a key element to developing an effective program. The following information should be collected as a part of a health promotion needs assessment: characteristics/demographics of those who will be participating in the program, the health education needs of the participants, hazard analysis issues relevant to the workplace, and the interests of the participants.

Planning/Development

Planning/development is the second of four phases that makes up this model. The information gathered in the assessment phase is used in the planning phase to develop the specific details of the program. Careful planning is an essential part in the successful implementation of any program. An advisory committee is often necessary to assist in the establishing of goals and objectives, as well as marketing strategies and a program budget. A timeline for implementation and completion of program activities is critical for keeping the program on track. When developing the actual content of the program, it is necessary to take into consideration the needs of the employees as well as the availability of resources. Finally, when developing any program, it is important that a means for evaluating is its effectiveness is established prior to implementation.

Implementation

Implementation is the third of four phases that makes up this model. This is the phase where the plan is put into action. Proper program development is the key for a smooth implementation. The follow-up and monitoring aspects of this phase are intended to make sure that the program is working as it should. Follow-up and monitoring activities include checking with employees to see if there are any questions or if information needs clarification. It also includes maintaining contact with participants (both short- and long-term) to assess their success in incorporating healthful choices into their lives.

Evaluation

Evaluation is the last of the four phases that makes up this model. It refers back to the goals and objectives that were established in the planning phase to see if the program did indeed do what was intended. There are three types of evaluation: process, impact, and outcome evaluation. Process evaluation looks at the actual process of conducting the program, including things such as materials used, resources available, and the space needed to conduct activities. Impact evaluation deals with whether or not short-term objectives were accomplished (i.e. smoking cessation, lower blood pressure, weight loss). Outcome evaluation, on the other hand, assesses the long-term effects of incorporating behavioral/lifestyle changes.

Delivery Methods for Health Promotion Educational Program

There are many different ways that a health promotion educational program can be presented to the target population. The **delivery method** that is chosen should coincide with the interests and abilities of those participating in the program. The assessment and planning phases of program development can help shed light on the optimal delivery methods for program activities. Some of the different methods that can be used in delivering a health promotion educational program include "On the Job Training" (OJT), distance learning, independent study, lectures, discussions, computer-based training, group exercises, demonstrations, or simulations.

Communication Methods

Some **traditional, nontraditional, and technology-based communication methods** that can be used in a health promotion program are as follows:

- **Traditional**: Announcements, written individual notices, bulletin board notices, pamphlets, payroll inserts, marquees and billboards, face-to-face individual sessions, group information sessions, audio presentations, audio-visual presentations, video presentations.
- **Nontraditional**: Information-based puzzles, self-quizzes, health risk appraisals, mail-requested vehicles, trigger cards, electronic bulletin boards, fax networks, online telephone support.
- **Technology-Based**: Electronic mail, proactive telephone contact, computer-based multimedia presentations, interactive voice response, tailored messaging, interactive information kiosk, internet websites, virtual reality applications, adaptive survey technology.

Knowles' Principles of Adult Education

The **four principles of adult education** (Knowles, 1984) are as follows:

1. **Independent learning** – The independence of adult learners is recognized and respected by giving them with self-directed activities.
2. **Previous experience** – The experiences of the participants is referred to and used as a base onto which new information is added.
3. **Readiness to learn** – Moments when participants are receptive to information (pregnancy, diagnosis with an illness, knowledge of someone affected by a disease) are utilized to the advantage of the instructor.
4. **Problem-oriented learning** - The specific concerns and problems of the participants are addresses, making the learning experience relevant and specific.

Principles of Epidemiology

Epidemiology

Epidemiology is defined as the study of the distribution and causes of disease and injury in the human population, as well as the application of this knowledge to control health problems. The basic underlying concept of any epidemiologic investigation is the idea that disease is caused by the interaction of several different factors and therefore cannot be pinned down to one cause. There are several different models that are used to describe this concept of "multiple causation," however they all incorporate the interaction between the host (human being and inherent factors such as age, genetics, health history), environment (external factors that influence host), and agent (factor necessary to produce a condition such as a virus, chemical, etc.).

Agent

The basic underlying concept of any epidemiologic investigation is the idea that disease is caused by the interaction of several different factors and therefore cannot be pinned down to one cause. There are several different models that are used to describe this concept of "multiple causation," however they all incorporate the interaction between the agent, host, and environment.

The term **agent**, as it is used in epidemiology, is the substance (virus, bacteria, chemical, allergen, etc.) that must be present in the host in order for a specific condition to occur. There are a number of different methods of used for the transmission of an agent to its host. For example, transmission of toxic substances can occur with the inhalation of toxic vapors. Infectious diseases are spread by various types of person-to-person contact such as sneezing or sexual intercourse or through indirect transmission such as a contaminated water supply.

Host Factors

The **host** is the living organism that is infected by the disease or condition. **Host factors** are those things that are specific to each individual and influence the likelihood that they will become infected with by agent (susceptibility). Host factors include age, gender, ethnicity, genetic profile, family health history, lifestyle risk factors, and health status.

Environmental Factors

Environmental factors are the external conditions (both physical and social) that can have an effect on the virulence of agent and/or the susceptibility of the host. Physical conditions include things such as water, temperature, elements, pollution, and industrial waste. Social conditions refer to the economic and political influences in society that can have an impact on the health of a population. Examples of social conditions that affect health include sanitation and hygiene, housing conditions, the availability of healthcare services, employment conditions, population growth, and literacy.

Measurement of Disease Frequency

Disease frequency is the most basic measure of the occurrence of a disease in a population. It is expressed as a rate that takes into consideration the size of the at-risk population and when the infection events occurred. Rates of disease are referred to as morbidity, while rates of death are called mortality. Mathematically, it is expressed as follows:

(Number of events/ Number of people at risk) x (population constant k)

The population constant (k) is incorporated to make it easier to compare different rates. Most statistics are reported per 100,000 people (population constant of 100,000).

EPIDEMIOLOGIC ANALYSIS

Once epidemiological data are collected, they must be **analyzed** so that they can provide information on disease risks and trends. To do this, the data are presented in a table indicating the presence of disease and exposure. The data are divided into four groups labeled a (number of individuals exposed who have the disease), b (number of individuals exposed who do not have the disease), c (number of individuals unexposed who have the disease), and d (number of individuals unexposed who do not have the disease). This information can then be combined in the following ways to provide the following specific information: the total number exposed (a + b), the total number unexposed (c + d), the total number with the disease (a + c), and the total number without the disease (b + d). Using these totals, relative risk (disease rate in exposed / disease rate in unexposed) is calculated as follows: (a/[a + b]) / (c/[c + d]).

SOURCES FOR DATA COLLECTION

Data used in epidemiologic studies come from many different **sources**. It is important that any data be accurate, therefore dependable sources of information must be found. There are several government offices that are responsible for gathering the data used in epidemiologic studies. The National Center for Health Statistics collects and analyzes health data including census information (births and deaths) and vital statistics. The Centers for Disease Control and Prevention collects demographic, clinical, and laboratory data on notifiable diseases (i.e. AIDS, diphtheria, malaria, sexually transmitted diseases, tetanus, and tuberculosis). The Bureau of Labor Statistics keeps an Occupational Injury and Classification System that is particularly useful in occupational health studies. Other useful sources of health information include hospital records, health records from physicians, insurance records, disease registries, health survey data, and occupational disease surveillance.

Education Topics and Barriers

Smoking Cessation Resources

Complementary therapies	Hypnosis: Breaks emotional attachment to smoking. Acupuncture: Reduces cravings and withdrawal symptoms. Meditation: Changes thought processes and behavior.
Stop smoking programs	The most successful programs usually require at least 4 sessions of 15 to 30 minutes and last ≥2 weeks or longer. "Quick fix" programs are less effective.
Telephone hotlines and help-lines	All states and the District of Columbia offer free telephone support to help people quit smoking. National helplines include: American Cancer Society: 1-800-227-2345 National Cancer Institute: 1-800-422-6237 National Quitline: 1-800-QUIT-NOW
Online support groups	Quitnet.com Quitsmokingjournals.com
Support groups	Numerous support groups are available, including: Nicotine Anonymous®, a 12-step national support program Smart Recovery®, an addiction recovery support group.
Family/Friends/Co-workers	A social support system is very important.

AIDS Education

Important elements of **AIDS education** include:

- Brief history of the disease: First case in Congo 1951, first US case 1981, first identified 1984, first FDA-approved treatment 1995, and home testing kits 2002.
- Nature of the disease, including infection stages (acute HIV infection, clinical latency, symptomatic AIDS) and common AIDS complications.
- Modes of transmission: Oral, anal, and vaginal sex as well as sharing of needles and contact with infected blood, semen, vaginal fluids, and breast milk.
- Prevention techniques, including safe sex practice (condom use) and safe needle use.
- At risk populations: multiple sex partners, males-having-sex with males, injection drug users, African Americans.
- Community resources for HIV testing.
- Legal and ethical issues: Information regarding rights to confidentiality and reporting requirements.
- Standard precautions to be used with contact with body fluids.
- Indications/Symptoms associated with HIV/AIDS.
- Available treatment options.
- Stigma and discrimination.

Barriers to Educational Process

Potential **barriers to the educational process** include:

- **Literacy**: Health literacy is the ability to obtain, understand, and consent to medical care, making informed healthcare decisions. Health literacy may be impacted by a number of factors, including lack of adequate education (low reading level), illiteracy, dementia, and learning disabilities. Those most vulnerable include the elderly, ethnic minorities, immigrants, and those with low income and/or chronic medical or physical health problems.
- **Language**: Language issues may arise when people speak no or limited English as well as when people are hearing or vision impaired. Foreign language or sign language interpreters may be necessary to ensure adequate communication. Readability (the grade level of material) is a concern when working with patients and families with limited English skills (or low literacy), and videos may be more effective than written materials. Some patients may have communication disorders, such as aphasia, which interferes with their ability to communicate or comprehend, and the assistance of a speech therapist may help to determine the most effective means of communication.

Education and Health Promotion Theory

Behavioral Theories as Related to Health Education and Promotion

Behavioral Management Theories

Two traditional behavioral management theories are Frederick Taylor's **scientific management theory** (1917) and Elton Mayo's **motivation theory** (1933):

- **Scientific management theory:** Management's role is to plan and control, identifying tasks and then assigning the best person to complete the tasks, utilizing both rewards and punishment as motivating forces. This theory puts the focus on the outcomes rather than on the individuals, but workers are often unmotivated with this structure.
- **Motivation theory:** This theory requires that managers take a more personal interest in the needs of workers. Mayo (in the Hawthorne experiment) found that workers responded positively to changes in the working environment and were motivated by increased managerial interest and involvement, team work, and improved communication between management and staff in which workers are consulted about decisions.

Operant Conditioning

B.F. Skinner developed the Theory of Radical Behaviorism based on the concept that behavior is dependent on the environment and reinforcement. Skinner believed that society influenced the individual and that behavior could be managed by **operant conditioning**. Skinner stated that the individual operates on the environment and encounters stimuli that bring forth a response. Those stimuli that increase the likelihood of a particular response are called reinforcers, and the goal of therapy is to find the appropriate stimuli to reinforce desired behavior. Both positive reinforcement in which a response is applied and negative reinforcement in which a response is removed are used to control and mold behavior. Skinner believed that aversive events (such as punishment) weakened behavior but that positive response was most effective. The most important factors in teaching an individual include providing feedback immediately, proceeding from simple to complex in small steps, and providing repetition and positive reinforcement.

Classical Conditioning

Pavlov developed the theory of **classical conditioning** with experiments on dogs. When presenting food to dogs (unconditioned stimulus), they began to salivate (unconditioned response). During Pavlov's experiments, he used a number of neutral stimuli (buzzers, light flashes) to determine if he could elicit salivation. He found that these stimuli by themselves did not, but if he paired a stimulus, such as a flashing light, with an unconditioned stimulus (food), the animal would eventually salivate in response to the flashing light (conditioned response), a learned behavior. Principles include:

- **Acquisition**: Time during which the unconditioned stimulus and conditioned stimulus are presented together (a gradual increase in learning occurs).
- **Second-order conditioning**: A neutral stimulus brings about the same conditioned response when presented with a conditioned stimulus (learning builds on previous steps).
- **Extinction**: If the conditioned stimulus (light) is presented repeatedly without the unconditioned stimulus (food), the conditioned response (learning) fades.
- **Spontaneous recovery**: After extinction, the conditioned response returns when presented with the conditioned stimulus (recovery of learning occurs).
- **Generalization**: Conditioned response occurs even with slight changes in the conditioned stimulus (building on previous learning).

Risk Assessment and Research

Health Risk Assessment

Health risk assessment is an organized and formal method of decreasing liability, financial loss, and risk or harm to patients, workers, or others by doing an assessment of risk and introducing risk management strategies. Much of risk management has been driven by the insurance industry in order to minimize costs, but quality management utilizes risk management as a method to ensure quality healthcare and process improvement as well as compliance. Identification of health risk is essential in developing strategies of health promotion. Steps include:

- **Risk identification** begins with an assessment of processes to identify and prioritize those that require further study to determine risk exposure.
- **Risk analysis** requires a careful documenting of process, utilizing flow charts, with each step in the process assessed for potential risks. This may utilize root cause analysis methods.
- **Risk prevention** involves instituting corrective or preventive processes. Responsible individual or teams are identified and trained.
- **Assessment/evaluation** of corrective/preventive processes is ongoing to determine if they are effective or require modification.

Need for Nursing Research

Because the field of nursing is a field where the information that is learned is applied in real-life situations that can affect the well-being of the patient, it is important to make sure that nurses have current information about illness, injury, diseases, and treatment options. Participating in research activities is one way that nurses and nursing information can remain current. There are several ways that a professional nurse can be involved in **research**. They can conduct literature reviews to stay up-to-date on topics relevant to their area of specialty; or they can participate in research investigation. The level of participation in research investigation can include development, design, or execution of research projects.

Research-Specific Terms

The definitions of **research-specific terms** are as follows:

- **Concept** – Observation-based ideas that are the building blocks of theories.
- **Theory** – An explanation of a fact or event.
- **Variable** –Something within an experiment that can have different values.
- **Attribute variable** – Variables that are inherent characteristics of the research subject (age, weight, health beliefs, etc.).
- **Independent variable** – Variable that is manipulated in an experiment with the expectation that it will have an effect on another variable.
- **Dependent variable** – Variable that is being assessed for changes based on manipulations of the independent variable.
- **Operational definition** – Details about how the dependent variable will be measured.
- **Extraneous variable** – Variables that are not under investigation but that can have an effect on the dependent variable. These variables need to be controlled so as not to incorrectly influence the results of the experiment.
- **Data** – Information collected from the experiment.

Qualitative Research

Qualitative research is different from the structured, numbers-oriented approach of quantitative research. In quantitative research, experiments are designed with goal of collecting numerical data. Qualitative research, on the other hand, is descriptive in nature, focusing on the different ways to describe and explain complex issues that cannot be numerically measured. There are different ways to collect the information that makes up qualitative research: description and interpretation, phenomenology (understanding of how people respond to and understand a particular phenomenon), and grounded theory (understanding of social and psychological experiences). While much of the research conducted in nursing is quantitative, there are plenty of applications of qualitative research as well (such as the ways people perceive and respond to health and safety issues).

Ethical Responsibility in Research

Although there are several **ethical issues** that come up when conducting occupational health research, they all fall under the umbrella of protection of the rights of the human subjects involved in research. These rights, which belong to all people involved in scientific research studies are as follows: The right to self-determination (not coerced into participating); the right to informed consent; the right to full disclosure; the right to privacy confidentiality, and anonymity; and the right to protection from harm. None of these rights should ever be compromised for the sake of research, regardless of the benefits.

Management Principles

Program Design

Manager Role of Occupational Health and Safety Nurse

The **occupational health and safety nurse** plays many roles within the health and safety program of a company. These roles were defined by the American Association of Occupational Health Nurses (AAOHN) in 1999 in conjunction with the standards of practice at that time (that have since been updated, but the roles remain relevant).

One of these is the role of the nurse as **manager**. As a manager, the occupational nurse provides the structure, organization, and guidance necessary to effectively administer the program. This aspect of the job entails the gathering of data about the worksite and workforce, and then using this data to plan the appropriate course of action, organizing personnel and necessary supplies, staffing, and the evaluation of both the program and the staff. In this capacity, the occupational health nurse is also responsible for providing health and safety reports to management.

Occupational Health and Safety Programs

Inputs

An **input** is anything that enters a system for processing. This can include both energy and information. Some of the inputs to an occupational health program include the culture, mission, and goals of an organization, as well as any work processes or procedures. Corporate culture and mission are an important part of an occupational health program because this ultimately sets the environmental controls and perceived importance of the workers' health and safety. The attitudes towards work processes and health and safety practices (at both a corporate and worker level) greatly determine the needs (or inputs) that an occupational health and safety program must address.

Throughputs

Throughputs are an intermediary stage. They include any action or procedure (also called an intervention) that changes the input, thus producing the final product. Some of the throughputs that are a part of an occupational health program are as follows: clinical analysis, surveillance programs and workplace walkthroughs, case management, employee counseling, decision making skills, occupational health policies, organizational policies and procedures, as well as training and research. Because the interventions that are a part of the throughput process are designed to meet the needs of the workers and organizational goals, it is important that the occupational health nurse accurately assesses these needs so as to maximize the throughput process.

Outputs

The ultimate goal of any occupational health program is healthy workers. More specifically, this goal is reflected in the **outputs** of the program. This final product of any system is called an output. Some of the typical outputs of an occupational health program are the prevention of illness and injury, the elimination of workplace hazards, and the overall improvement of worker health and safety. Each of these outputs is accomplished through changes in behavior (both occupational and non-occupational) and the implementation of hazard protection policies. The organization often realizes overall improvement due to positive outputs. In the case of occupational health, this can come in the form of the reduction of healthcare costs, a reduction in absenteeism, and an increase in productivity.

Feedback

Feedback mechanisms consist of any number of processes or procedures that exist for the purpose of evaluating the output results and the process that created them. They exist for the purpose making the system well organized and effective. This is an important aspect of any system because effectiveness is measured by a comparison of the outputs to the objectives of the program and it is in through the feedback process that program deficiencies are often discovered.

Development

A **system** is made up of **four major parts.** These are inputs, throughputs, outputs, and feedback mechanisms:

1. An **input** is anything that enters a system for processing. This can include both energy and information.
2. **Throughputs** are an intermediary stage. They include any action or procedure that changes the input, thus producing the final product.
3. This final product is called an **output**.
4. **Feedback mechanisms** consist of any number of processes or procedures that exist for the purpose of evaluating the output results and the process that created them.

It is in this way that the entire system is made more efficient and effective. The occupational health and safety system fits within this general system model. One example of this is a production process as an input, the ergonomic standards as the throughput, with the output being a healthy employee. The feedback mechanisms in this system would be worksite and employee evaluations.

Population Health and Healthcare Trends

One such external influence is population health and **healthcare trends**. The overall health and healthcare practices of the population are often reflected in the workforce because the workforce usually comes from this population. Any occupational health and safety program should be tailored to the specific part of the population that is represented in the workforce.

This is because different populations have different healthcare concerns. For example, prenatal care, maternity leave, and childcare would not be concerns of an elderly population.

Legislation, Regulation, and Politics

Legislation, regulation, and politics are some of these external influences. Over the years, laws and regulations have been instituted that have a direct impact on occupational health programs. Two that are well known are the Americans with Disabilities Act (ADA) and the Family Medical Leave Act (FMLA). It is imperative that all relevant laws and regulations be taken into consideration when developing any occupational health program. Keeping a program up-to-date may require the adjustment and/or expansion of program objectives and goals, as well as an increase in financial allocation to the program to help institute and maintain the mandated programs and requirements.

Technology

Another external influence is **technology**. Technology can have both a positive or negative effect on occupational health. On one hand, it may result in an increase in production that can be physically tasking to the employee or cause physical stresses that result in accident or injury to the employee. An example of this is the use of computers and the development of carpel tunnel syndrome. On the other hand, it can allow for the redesign and implementation of safer and more efficient work processes. New technology should always be analyzed and monitored for the potential for worker harm.

ECONOMICS

The final external influence is **economics**. The economics of a company can influence many aspects of the company. It has the potential to affect the confidence and efficiency of the workforce. When the economic outlook of a company is poor, it is can necessitate layoffs of reductions in the workforce which, in turn, can result in economic difficulties for employees. One of the difficulties that employees may face during economic hardship is an increase in healthcare costs. By implementing a cost-effective occupational health program, a company can ease the burden of the cost of healthcare. Some of the services that an occupational health program can provide to this end include health promotion and education programs, health screening procedures, and on-site primary care services.

Program Evaluation/Assessment

Culture Assessment in Occupational Health Nursing

Power Culture

There are several types of **organizational cultures**, one of which is **power culture**. Power culture refers to an organizational culture that relies on an imbalance of power to run the organization where one or more individuals hold power over others. This imbalance of power usually has a hierarchical structure and leaders are an integral part in maintaining this structure. Because this type of culture is power-based, there is a potential for those who have all of the power to use it for personal gain or to instill fear in those beneath them.

Role Culture

Role culture refers to an organizational culture that relies on the responsibilities of every individual within the workplace to maintain order and productivity. This is not a hierarchical structure with one individual at the top managing everyone else. Instead, all workers have an understanding of their role and within the workplace, and routinely perform the responsibilities associated with this role without much control or oversight. This type of organizational culture requires a workplace with a routine in place and a workforce that is willing to adhere to it.

Achievement Culture

Behaviors are often learned while working within the organization, but can come from outside sources as well. This can be the case if the workforce comes from one population group. An **achievement culture** refers to an organizational culture that relies on the worker's job satisfaction to maintain order and productivity. It requires a style of management that focuses on employee morale and promotes excitement for the work process.

Support Culture

Support culture is a type of organizational culture that is interested in meeting the needs of the individual with the intent of maintaining accord within the workplace. In this type of organizational culture, there is less of a focus on goals and mission statements, and more importance placed on trust and harmony between workers.

Effects of Organizational Culture on Decision-Making Process

Each of the different organizational cultures has a different view on the **decision-making process.** This can, in turn, have an effect on the way an occupational health program is run. For example, power culture limits decisions to those that hold all of the power; role culture divides decision-making between workers depending on their role relevant responsibilities; achievement culture focuses on making decisions that build employee morale; and support culture focuses on decisions that maintain peace and harmony within the workforce.

Culture Assessment of Organizations

Assessment of Organizational Politics

An **assessment of politics** with a company sheds light on the type of power structure in place, who is responsible for most of the decisions, how the decision-making process is distributed amongst the workforce, and the number of resources that are available for distribution to particular programs. While organizational politics is not an important part of actual health and safety, it can play role in the degree of support for an occupational health and safety program, the availability of supplies and funds, as well as attitudes towards safety and compliance.

Assessment of Organization's Formal Structure

An **assessment of an organization's formal structure** is a part of the culture assessment of an organization. An understanding of the formal structure provides insight into how an organization is managed, the hierarchy of responsibility, as well as its goals and mission. By having an understanding of the formal structure of the organization, the occupational health nurse can design a program that fits within the management and policy-making confines of the company.

Assessment of Organization's Formal and Informal Communication Structures

Formal communication structures are all of the methods of relaying information that are authorized by management including include memos, meeting, and evaluations. There is often an established form and format for these modes of communication.

Informal communication, on the other hand, refers to the unofficial passing on of information. These types of communication structures are casual, with little or no format, and are often not authorized by management. Both forms of communication affect the way that information is passed on to others and interpreted.

Leadership Styles and Behaviors

The **style of leadership** that is employed at an organization often has a historical precedent, with new leaders exhibiting the same ideals and behaviors as their predecessors. This is what allows a company to maintain a particular mission over long periods of time. The style of leadership can also affect the productivity of the workforce due to the policies, procedures, and values that are established and upheld from one leader to the next.

Assessment of Organization's Work Environment

Organizational culture encompasses all of the ideals and behaviors that that unify the workforce to a common goal. An assessment of an **organization's work environment** is a part of the culture assessment of an organization. This plays a direct role in any occupational health program because work environment can greatly affect the physical and mental well-being of the workforce. In fact, environmental health is one of the focus areas of an occupational health and safety program. Aspects of the work environment that are important to assess include workplace hygiene, safety, productivity, and stress.

Image and Status Symbols Within the Organization

Image and status are directly related to power, however, this power does not necessary correlate with the leaders of the organization. The location of parking spaces, the type of office or work environment, and even the hours that a person works can all be seen as status symbols that influence the image of both the worker and the organization as a whole.

Organizational Culture

Positional Power

Workplace power can have either a positive or negative effect on the workforce and this greatly depending on the degree of importance that is placed on the workers and their needs. There are three different types of power and these are categorized based on the sources of the power. Positional power is one type of power. This type of power usually comes from an individual's position within the hierarchy of the company; however, it can also be based on things such as the leader's ability to compensation the workers, the control of knowledge that is considered significant, or fear of retribution or punishment.

Personal Power

Personal power is one type of power and it relies on the personal characteristics of the individual. There are two types of personal power. The first is expert power. It is based on an individual's possession of a talent or skill that is considered important. In this type of power, the individual is valued for their expertise. The second type of personal power is referent power. It is founded in how well an individual is liked and respected by their coworkers.

Interpersonal Power

Interpersonal power is one type of power. It comes from an individual's connection to others that are considered important, either inside or outside of the organization. The significance of the individual is dependent not on personal characteristics, but on one's associations with others.

Communication/Performance

Management Skill Levels

The three **management skill levels** that are important to an individual's role as manager are as follows:

1. **Technical Skills** – The understanding and ability to use all of the equipment and procedures necessary to complete a particular job or work process.
2. **Interpersonal Skills** – The understanding of behavior, motivational strategies, and effective communication techniques as they relate to establishing and maintaining relationships in the workplace.
3. **Conceptual Skills** – The ability to understand, analyze, and apply complicated ideas and theories to tasks and processes within the workplace.

There are **three management skill levels** that exist within the manager role of an occupational health nurse. These are technical skills, interpersonal skills, and conceptual skills. All three of these skills are necessary components of successful managers. The relative importance and degree of use, however, depends on the manager's role within the structure of the company as well as each individual management situation. Managers that exist at a higher level within a company rely less on technical skills and more on conceptual. If one is responsible for training new employees, both technical and interpersonal skills are used to a greater degree than conceptual. Regardless of the situation and appropriate skill mix, it is important that managers have the knowledge and the ability to use all three skill levels as well as an understanding of how they interrelate.

Difficult Communication Behaviors

There are times when an occupational health nurse may run into **difficult communication** behaviors in employees that will need to be addressed in order to run an effective occupational health program. These behaviors include hostility, complaining, unresponsiveness, and negativity. When these types of communication behaviors are encountered, it is important that the occupational health nurse utilize the communication skills necessary to compose, redirect the employee's behavior with the goal of discussing and resolving the issue at hand. Some of the tactics that one can employ include removing the employee from the immediate work environment, listening to the employee's complaints and exploring possible solutions, as well as using open-ended questions to promote the expression of feelings and concerns.

Types of Communication

There are **three basic types of communication**. These are vertical communication, lateral (also called horizontal) communication, and informal communication:

- **Vertical communication** is hierarchically based, moving up and down from the employees up to managers and supervisors or the other way around. Implicit in this type of communication is the freedom of employees to communicate their thoughts and desires.
- **Lateral communication** moves between departments at the same level. This is not a hierarchical form of communication; instead, communication occurs between managers or between coworkers. Both vertical and lateral communication is necessary parts of a successful organization.

- **Informal communication** is the third type of communication. This is usually referred to as the "grapevine" and although it is not typically a management-approved form of communication, it is quite common in the workplace and thus should be recognized as one of the ways that employees get information. However, because there is no means for regulation or responsibility within this type of communication, the information that is passed on is not always accurate.

Decision-Making Processes

Effective decision-making is an important part of the manager role of an occupational health nurse. The decision-making process entails a series of educated, well-planned steps that lead to rational, problem solving results. Within an occupational health program, there are several tools and techniques available to personnel to facilitate the decision-making process. These include activities such as brainstorming, decision trees, program evaluation and review techniques (PERT), Delphi methods, forecasting, and simulated computer applications. There are times when the occupational health nurse may make decisions independent of others within the organization, but more often than not, the decision-making process is a group activity where many individuals are involved including doctors, nurses, safety personnel, employees, supervisors, and upper management.

Steps

The **decision-making process consists of 5 steps**. They are as follows:

1. **Identify the problem** – Identify the problem and gather as much information and data as possible so that it can be fully understood and analyzed.
2. **Determine courses of action** – Delineate as many different ways to solve the problem as possible. Provide the pros and cons for each possible course of action.
3. **Decide on a course of action** – Taking into consideration the pros and cons of each course of action, the most appropriate one should be selected.
4. **Implement the decision** – Once a decision has been made, it must be implemented. This step requires a great deal of organization and communication to be effective.
5. **Evaluate the decision results** – The effectiveness of the decision should be evaluated. It is important that enough time has passed to allow for the most accurate evaluation possible. If it is determined that the decision is not working, it should be adjusted accordingly.

Managerial Process

PLANNING

There are two basic **types of planning** and both require conceptual thinking skills:

- The first is **strategic planning**, which is long range planning that is more generic and less specific.
- The second is **operational planning**, which is a specific, short-term type of planning.

In any type of planning, it is important to understand and address the organization's mission, strengths and weaknesses, values, goals, and objectives.

VISION AND MISSION

The **vision** of a company depicts its image as it relates to the goals and plans for the future. A **mission statement** defines an organization's reason for existence. Both the vision and mission of a company direct the goals and objectives that are established during the planning phase of the managerial process. The goals and objectives of each department must relate back to the vision and mission. However, it is not just a company that can have a vision and mission, but the departments within the company and individual personnel often have one as well. This is particularly the case for an occupational health program. In fact, because an occupational health program has so many roles within a company, without a vision or mission, it could easily become unfocused and ineffective.

GOALS AND OBJECTIVES

During the planning phase of the managerial process, it is important to establish **goal and objectives**. These goals and objectives should refer back to the vision and mission of both the company and the program. Goals are statements that provide information regarding the overall ambitions of a company, department, or individual.

Once goals are established, concrete steps that can be taken to reach these goals are outlined. These steps are called objectives. Both goals and objects are integral parts of the planning process. Without objectives, goals are not often met. Without goals, objectives are unfocused. All goals and objectives should be periodically evaluated to assess the success of achievement and adjusted as necessary.

BUSINESS PROPOSALS AND PLANS

As a part of the planning aspect of the managerial process, an occupational health nurse is required to **develop business proposals** and **plans**. The purpose of any business proposal/plan is to secure support for a project. This support can come in the form of general approval, funding, equipment, or personnel. All business proposals/plans follow a similar format, regardless of their ultimate goal. This is so that proposals from different areas of a company can be compared and assessed for relative importance. Because the availability of funds is often limited, it is important that any business proposal/plan provide a justification for support.

The basic **parts of a business proposal/plan** are as follows:

- Title Page: Title, author, date of submission, date of implementation.
- Project/Executive Summary: Overview of project.
- Table of Contents: Reference page numbers to each section.
- Introduction: Company's or program's goals and objectives.
- Project Description: Description of the purpose of the project.
- Rationale/Identification of Need: Justification for need.
- Alternative Approaches: Problems and issues and how they will be addressed.
- Operational Plan: Description of how the project will be carried out.
- Marketing Plan: Intended audience and how the project will be brought to them.
- Financial Plan: Budget that delineates all project costs.
- Evaluation Plan: Project assessment.
- Appendices: All necessary supporting documents.

Financial Management

Planning, financial management, organizing, staffing, directing, and evaluating are the six major functions of the managerial process. The **financial management function** entails financial planning, budgeting, and identification of resources. The financial manager is responsible for keeping track of all of the monetary aspects of an organization or program. This includes keeping track of income and expenses, keeping all necessary financial documentation using a well-organized system, suggesting cost reduction strategies, as well as explaining the budget and spending to upper management. With increases in healthcare costs, this aspect of occupational health nursing has become increasingly important. Indeed, a major function of any occupational health program is the cost-effective provision of health services.

Budget Preparation Process

As a part of the financial aspect of the managerial process, managers must be able to draft a **budget**. A budget provides financial information on how resources will be allocated over a specific period of time. A budget can be created for a company, department, or project. An effective budget accurately anticipates future costs. There are two basic kinds of budgets that an occupational health manager needs to be familiar with: operating budget and capital expense budget. An operating budget provides information about the everyday expenses incurred in the operations of a company, department, or project. Information such as previous budgets, current goals and objectives, as well as anticipated needs future growth are all taken into consideration when drafting an operating budget. A capital expense budget is a long-term planning tool that looks at the financial aspects of larger projects typically dealing with expansion. These are usually expensive propositions that must be assessed for importance based on financial impact, investment recovery time, and need relative to other large-scale projects.

Organization

Without **organization**, nothing would get past the planning stage. As an organizer, the occupational health nurse provides an official structure to the program that allows for the establishment and meeting of objectives, as well as the obtaining of resources necessary for program success. Some of these resources include a physical space in which to conduct activities, as well as the necessary equipment, supplies, and personnel. The overall purpose of any organizing activity within an occupational health and safety program is the provision of a safe and healthy work environment.

Span of Management

Span of management (also called span of control) is a part of the organizational side of the managerial process. It deals with the relationship between the manager and workers. Specifically, it describes the number of workers under the control of the manager. When determining the span of control of a manager, it is important to assess the number of personnel that can be effectively managed by a particular manager. This can vary within a company, with the primary factors that influence it being the type of work, education and abilities of the workers, the number of duties of the manager, and the physical space necessary for the processes being managed. Time and span of control are inversely proportional, with any task or management process that requires a greater input of time decreasing a manager's effective span of control.

Centralization vs. Decentralization

The degree of **centralization versus decentralization** of management responsibility is one part of the organizational aspect of the managerial process. A company that is highly centralized is one where one top official (usually the chief executive officer) makes most of the decisions. This style of management reduces the need for planning and critical thinking at lower levels. Decentralization refers to the degree to which the decision-making process is spread throughout the company. In this style of management control is not concentrated at the top, but divided between lower managers and even workers. In order for decentralization to be effective, managers and workers must not only be reliable, but their supervisors must also support and believe in their skills and capabilities.

Delegation

One part of the organizational aspect of the managerial process is the ability to **delegate responsibilities** to others. Delegation refers to transferring a task or responsibility from a member of management to one of the workers. It relies on the skills and abilities of the worker to perform tasks that are not necessarily a typical part of their job description. In order for delegation to be effective, the worker must be officially assigned the responsibility to complete the task with the authority to make the necessary decisions. Additionally, the worker must accept that they have a responsibility to successfully complete the project as well as the consequences for the outcome.

Policies and Procedures

Policies and procedures are developed as a tool to support the hierarchical organization of a company. Any policies or procedures should be focused on meeting the goals and objectives of the organization. Policies usually apply to an entire company. They are typically defined in a policy manual and are geared towards addressing potential problems, defining authority and limits of control, as well as delineating job-specific functions. Procedures, on the other hand, tend to be more localized and department-specific than policies. They give details about detailed actions and define the steps necessary to complete particular activities or work processes. Both policies and procedures should be assessed regularly for relevance and updated as necessary. Any updates to policies or procedures should be provided to all personnel.

Position/Job Description

A **position/job description** provides information about the responsibilities associated with a specific job. Job descriptions are used to help when recruiting and interviewing new employees. They also provide a standard of comparison for conducting performance evaluations. The typical parts of a job description include the job title, a brief summary of the position, the span of control, a list of expectations and responsibilities, as well as a list of the necessary qualifications (knowledge, skills, education, and experience). Any responsibilities included in a job description should be listed in order of importance with the key duties associated with the position clearly described. Job descriptions must be accurate and up to date, with the date of the last revision noted. They should also be regularly assessed for relevance and updated as necessary.

STAFFING

The **staffing function** of the managerial process involves the recruitment, screening, and selection of personnel necessary to meet organizational a plans and objectives, as well as establishment and management of work schedules. This is a particularly important function because of its direct link to the overall success and productivity of the company. Without well-chosen employees, goals and objectives are not met, program plans are not put into action, and the growth of the organization is ultimately stalled.

RECRUITMENT

Some different methods of providing potential new employees with job information include employee referrals, word of mouth, advertising, disseminating **recruitment** literature, posters, providing information at career days or job fairs, utilizing placement services, holding company open houses, as well as the connections established at conventions and meetings. Before beginning recruitment procedures, it is necessary to review and update the job description so that it is complete and accurate. When conducting any recruitment activity, it is important to meet necessary equal employment opportunity requirements.

COORDINATION OF WORK SCHEDULES

The staffing function of the managerial process involves the recruitment, screening, and selection of personnel necessary to meet organizational a plans and objectives, as well as establishment and **coordination of work schedules.** There is no standard for determining the number of employees necessary to complete a task. This greatly depends on the nature of the job and the abilities of employees and should be determined on a case-by-case basis. When establishing a work schedule, one must assess the job and determine the number of workers needed. It is also necessary to know the availability of personnel. Activities such as special training programs, vacation schedules, absenteeism, shift rotation, and special needs staff all potentially restrict the availability of workers. Thus, it may be necessary to periodically hire temporary employees help to meet staffing requirements.

PERSONNEL DEVELOPMENT

The **personnel development** of workers and managers is an important part of the staffing process. It provides workers with the education and ability essential for professional growth while at the same time providing managers with an educated and self-assured workforce. Staffing development activities include (but are not limited to) orientations, mentorships, skill checklists, internships, in-service education, supplementary courses, conferences, seminars, and journal/book clubs. It is important that managers support workers in personnel development activities by allowing and encouraging them to take the time to participate, as well as allocating finances for these activities in plans and budgets.

DIRECTING

The **directing function** of the managerial process deals with managing, communicating, and guiding employees. The amount of direction necessary depends on the factors such as the education, abilities, experience, and motivational qualities of both the individual employee and the group with which they are associated. Ultimately, all direction provides individuals with an understanding of what they are expected to accomplish and how they are supposed to do it. It is important in the directing aspect of the managerial process, not to over-direct or micromanage. This can negatively affect the workforce and workplace productivity. For this reason, the ability to understand and work with employees as well as excellent communication skills are indispensable qualities of an effective director.

Guidance

The directing function of the managerial process deals with managing, communicating, and guiding employees. The **guidance** aspect of the managerial process occurs when a new job or task is at hand and the manager needs to assess and select the best employee for the job. It is particularly important when employees volunteer for assignments for which they do not have much experience. It is up to the manager to review the job qualifications and skills of these workers and guide them to the most suitable job. As a director that needs to provide guidance to employees, a manager must be aware of the technical requirements of a job and be willing to provide the necessary education and training activities to allow workers to advance and remain competitive within their field.

Communication

A manager must be aware of the different types of **communication** (vertical, later, and informal), and know how to take this information and apply it to employee relationships. There are often situations where workers are troubled, angry, or speaking negatively of the company or workplace. These types of attitudes can quickly have a negative effect on the rest of the workforce, so it is imperative that a manager deals with it in a swift and appropriate manner. The goal is to provide the best work environment possible while maintaining worker productivity.

Change Management

Quite often, **changes** will occur in the workplace and it is important that a manager attempts to control these changes as much as possible. Ideally, change within the workplace should be planned and organized so as to provide the workforce with a stable work environment. Stability provides an optimal setting for accepting and handling change. There are three phases of change: unfreezing or stopping of the status quo with the understanding that there is a need for change, moving towards a new system through investigating possible solutions and plans for change, and refreezing the change process by accepting a change as normal and incorporating it into the status quo. Because change can lead to feelings of fear or uncertainty, a manager must be willing and able to deal with employee concerns before any change is instituted. This will help make the process of acceptance and integration as smooth as possible.

Evaluation

The **evaluating function** of the managerial process is a key part in determining the effectiveness of the program. No program or plan can be implemented without an evaluation step. Not only should programs be evaluated for efficacy, but employee performance should also be evaluated. It is through evaluation that problems are identified and corrected, programs and plans are adjusted, and the overall quality of the program is monitored. Some of the methods used for evaluation include setting performance standards, quality measurements, and quality control.

Resistance to Change

Strategies to Reduce Worker Resistance

Change can lead to feelings of fear or uncertainty, leading to a **resistance to change.** There are several strategies that can be employed to reduce worker resistance to change. By understanding these strategies, a manager can be ready and able to deal with employee concerns before any change is instituted, making the process of acceptance and integration as smooth as possible. Some of the strategies that can be employed by a manager to reduce worker resistance to change include (but are not limited to) involving worker in the process of investigating and planning for change, attempt to institute change first with those that are most likely to accept it, make sure the process of change is gradual, communicate changes clearly and accurately, be able to recognize those that are likely to resist change and identify the reasons for resistance, and allow individuals to accept change naturally and without force.

Influential Factors

There are several **factors that influence resistance to change**. By understanding these factors, a manager can be ready and able to deal with employee concerns before any change is instituted making the process of acceptance and integration as smooth as possible. These factors include (but are not limited to) threats to a worker's position within a company or job security, fear of making a mistake, unwanted pressure from the company or other workers, conflicts with personal goals and interests, breaking of traditions, and threats to an individual's feeling of power or confidence.

Quality Control/Assurance

Quality Assurance

Quality assurance programs are instituted within an occupational health program to improve the quality of healthcare, reduce costs, and provide a means for self-assessment and regulation. A measurable means of assessing the quality of care is necessary for any quality assurance program to be a success. This requires setting professional standards and comparing actual performance to these standards. These standards are most often set by the relevant professional society. The overall purpose of any quality assurance program is a dedication to providing quality services. Some of the most common methods used for quality assurance include audits, peer reviews, and quality circles.

Approaches to Quality Assurance Evaluation

There are **three major approaches** that form the basis for the evaluative mechanisms in quality assurance: structure, process, and outcome. The **evaluative elements** for each approach are as follows:

- **Structure** – the place where services are provided, values and mission of the organization, goals and objectives, human resources, financial resources, operational resources.
- **Process** – Management of services, decision making processes, collaboration between relevant personnel, actions and interventions, monitoring and evaluation, records and reports.
- **Outcome** – Goals are achieved, ordinances and recommendations are adhered to, ability to elicit positive changes, improved knowledge and skills base, satisfaction of recipients of service.

Practice Standards

Practice standards are developed by professional organizations as a means of regulating the quality of the services rendered within that field. As defined by the American Nurses Association (ANA), standards describe the responsibilities and obligations of those in the nursing profession. They are used in determining professional accountability, as well as a way to assess quality of care and services. ANA standards are generic, applying to all types of nursing. They are divided into two categories. The first are standards of care and focus on the ability of a nurse to do their job in a complete and accurate manner. The second are standards of professional performance and deal with the way that a nurse performs their job. In a sense, standards of care are quantitatively based and standards of professional performance are qualitatively based. Because standards are based on the ideals and ethics of the profession, they tend not to change over time.

PROFESSIONAL PRACTICE ACTIVITIES

Quality assurance programs in healthcare are designed to improve the quality of care while at the same time reduce healthcare costs. Models are developed and used when evaluating healthcare. **The Marker Umbrella Model for Quality Assurance (1987)** outlines nine activities that constitute professional practice. They are as follows:

1. Establishment of standards for professional practice.
2. Credentialing (licensure, performance monitoring, certification, and testing).
3. Continuing education.
4. Performance appraisals that are compared to established standards.
5. Audit procedures and data collection.
6. Monitoring that is a quick check of quality of care.
7. Ongoing problem identification and monitoring.
8. Resource utilization monitoring.
9. Continuous risk management.

QUALITY CIRCLES

A **quality circle** is one approach to quality assurance. It is a small group of employees (usually 5 to 10) that meets on a regular basis with the intention of the assessment, identification, and solving of issues and problems in the workplace. Once a problem or issue is identified, the group attempts to identify the root cause of the problem and suggests solutions. The solutions are presented to management for approval and then implemented by the group. The most important part of the entire process is evaluation of the implemented solution for effectiveness. Since the group is made up of employees, employee participation and feedback are at the heart of this approach to quality assurance.

QUALITY MANAGEMENT

Quality management (or continuous quality improvement) expands upon quality assurance principles by focusing on continuous improvement. The overall goal of quality management is to "do the right thing right the first time, on time, and all the time," and has the goal of continuous improvement. It emphasizes employee satisfaction through addressing problems within the workplace. This is not an approach where workers are kept happy through rewards, but through the establishment of a consistently improving, well-managed workplace that does not overlook the worker's issues or problems. In following quality management protocols, a company is taking a preventative approach to managing workers and the workplace.

BENCHMARKING

Benchmarking (comparing an organization's efforts with those of an external source or internal data) is especially important in compliance efforts to show where the organization is currently, the standard to which the comparison is made, and the organizational goal. Benchmark data is available from many sources including internal data, State Boards of Health, CMS, Hospital Compare website, professional organizations (such as the Society for Thoracic Surgeons), the Institute for Healthcare Improvement (IHI), and accreditation agencies (such as the Joint Commission). Benchmarking may be used to justify budgeting, to target interventions, and to ensure that an organization is meeting industry standards. Benchmarking data should be made widely available within an organization, such as on an organization dashboard, so that staff members are reminded of goals and can assess progress toward meeting these goals. These dashboards should also include information about incidents and areas of particular risk within the organization. Steps to effective benchmarking include choosing the industry standard and benchmarking standard with which to compare, identifying goals, selecting metrics, collecting and analyzing data, and assessing the data for process improvement.

Advantages of Quality Management

There are specific **advantages** that can be realized with the implementation of a quality management approach to running the workplace. These include (but are not limited to) an increase in the quality of work and productivity with a simultaneous decrease in the need to repeat work, a savings of time and money, an improvement in employee morale, as well as a decrease in employee turnover and recruitment costs.

Basic Services

A health assessment, monitoring, and surveillance program is a critical part of any occupational health program. While this program can incorporate many different health professionals (nurse, doctor, safety officer), it is often the occupational health nurse that is responsible for its implementation and management. Thus, it is important to understand the **basic services** that any health assessment, monitoring, and surveillance program should offer. They include the gathering and storage of worker health and safety information, job process analyses as a way to determine the effects of a job on the workforce, appropriate placement of workers within the company, occupational and non-occupational health and safety promotion and education programs, assessment of worker current health status (particularly for infection with communicable diseases), implementation and oversight of relevant hazard control strategies, compliance with mandatory programs, and worker rehabilitation programs.

Health Assessment and Surveillance

Health/Medical Surveillance Program

Health/medical surveillance programs are instituted when employees have the potential to be exposed to work-related health hazards and/or they are considered high risk for developing related negative health effects. The level to which a health/medical surveillance program is executed depends on the types of hazards to which employees may be exposed and the standards established by regulatory organizations such as OSHA or the National Institute for Occupational Safety and Health (NIOSH). Employees that are considered high risk must be assessed at a minimum of one a year. This assessment consists of a hazard-specific health history, physical exam, and tests.

Considerations for Development

When developing a health/medical surveillance program, there are several pieces of **information that should be taken into consideration**. It is important to have a complete understanding of population at risk. This includes assessing both health and demographic information. It is also necessary to have a full knowledge and understanding of workplace hazards and their potential negative health effects. Using all of this information, the occupational health nurse must establish a protocol of surveillance activities, tests, and data interpretation. Any Health/medical surveillance program must be in compliance with OSHA health and safety regulations.

Environmental Monitoring

Environmental monitoring is one aspect of a health/medical surveillance program. While worksite walk-throughs are usually the biggest part of an occupational health and safety program, regular environmental monitoring is also important. This type of monitoring assesses overall exposure levels in the environment and is used to detect environmental exposures that have the possibility to cause negative health effects to workers, but the levels are not high enough to be easily noticed. If contaminants are discovered, the amount of risk is determined by comparing the measurements to environmental exposure limits.

Symptoms That Trigger Health Surveillance Testing

Some of the **signs and symptoms of occupational exposure** to hazardous substances include (but are not limited to) headache, dizziness, drowsiness, nausea, and vomiting. If workers complain of any of these symptoms, occupational health and safety personnel should immediately begin surveillance testing of the area that includes ALL workers who are at risk, regardless of symptoms.

Health/Medical Surveillance Program

Physical Examinations

Physical examinations are one of the surveillance activities that can be instituted to help detect negative the health effects associated with exposure to a toxic substance or environmental hazard. They should be conducted by qualified health professionals that have an understanding of the stresses and hazards specific to the work environment. If the work environment necessitates the institution of a health/medical surveillance program, a physical exam can help identify non-work-related health conditions that could be made worse by an occupational exposure. One common condition exacerbated by occupational exposure is asthma.

Frequency of Examinations

Any examination must be conducted at a point where negative effects can be detected, but early enough to catch any health problems before they become severe. This means that they should be conducted on a **periodic, yet regular basis**. Because everyone can respond differently to an exposure, it is the responsibility of the occupational health and safety professional to be aware of all of the signs and symptoms of exposure and perform an examination as soon as they are observed.

Biological and Environmental Monitoring

Biological and environmental monitoring are both ways to assess the amount of exposure to workers as a part of a health/medical surveillance program. Biological monitoring provides occupational health professionals with information on the dose of a chemical within a worker, while environmental monitoring provides information on the levels of the chemical in the environment. Because biological monitoring is an indicator of the actual amount absorbed by the worker, it is a more accurate gauge of the potential toxic effect than a measurement of the amount of toxin in the environment. Biological monitoring also takes into consideration extraneous information such as route of exposure, source of exposure, and the use of personal protective devices. Environmental monitoring only provides information about the working environment.

Media

Biological monitoring is a commonly used assessment activity within a health/medical surveillance program. Several **different media** are used to assess the amount of toxin in a person's system: blood, urine, and exhaled air are the most common. Urine is the favored medium because it is noninvasive and it can be used to detect many different kinds of exposures. However, it is not always the most appropriate medium. Thus, when deciding what tests to issue, occupational health professionals must take into consideration additional information such as route of exposure, source of exposure, and the use of personal protective devices.

Variations in Test Results

Biological monitoring measures the presence of toxins and/or their by-products within the workers. Because it is a measurement of the amount of toxin that an individual has actually absorbed, it is important to conduct any biological monitoring tests at times when a substance is likely to be detected such as when a work shift is over. If tests are conducted at the start of a shift, they may not be sensitive enough to detect substances absorbed the previous day. There is always the potential for **variations** in the test results due to both work- and non-work-related factors. Some of these factors include diet, medications, alcohol consumption, cigarette smoking, time of specimen collection, and specimen contamination.

Biological Exposure Indices

Once tests are conducted, it is necessary to analyze and interpret the results. Common tools for this are **Biological Exposure Indices (BEI's).** They provide healthcare professionals with a measurement to which the results of biological monitoring tests can be compared and understood. If BEI's are not available, results can be compared to dose-response relationships or environmental levels to estimate the toxic effect. It is important to note that BEI's are warnings of exposure and not an indication of the negative effects of a substance.

Interpretation of Collected Data

The data collected as a part of a health/medical surveillance program must first be analyzed before it can be **interpreted** and understood. There are many different methods of data analysis, each focusing on determining the statistical value of the data. Regardless of the methods used, the data should always be interpreted in relation to the results expected in a healthy, unexposed population that is equivalent to the worker population being assessed.

Baseline Examinations

Any time that an individual is in a work environment that may require health/medical surveillance, it is important that a **baseline examination** be conducted that includes a complete medical history, physical exam, and relevant tests. A baseline examination will provide the occupational health professional with a reference point for future exams. Because of this, it is important that the tests that are selected to be a part of the exam are specific, accurate, and reliable enough to be used for future comparisons.

Plan of Action if Test Results Exceed Threshold Levels

If the test results from a health/medical surveillance exam **exceed established threshold levels,** further action is necessary. The results must be confirmed and assessed for accuracy. If necessary, the relevant specialist should be consulted to assure the proper reading of test results. If abnormal test results are confirmed, the potential causes must be identified and steps taken for remediation. The employee should always be referred to a physician or specialist for an official diagnosis and to get information about treatment options.

Notifying Employees of Exam Results

When any type of monitoring activity or test is deemed necessary, it is important to **notify the employee** of the results. This should be done in writing, by the appropriate healthcare professional. This notification should include the following information: the actual test results and their implications, the risks that come with exposure to the hazard, steps necessary to eliminate or reduce exposure, medical referral/follow-up, the necessity for future testing and monitoring, as well as important legal issues such as workers' compensation rights/benefits.

Necessary Steps if Adverse Health Effects Are Detected

If control measures are not possible or effective, employees at risk for exposure should be removed from the environment. In the event that the negative health effect limits the worker's ability to perform their previous job, they should then be placed in a different work environment/job.

Follow-Up Steps After Modifications

Health/medical surveillance activities focus on monitoring individuals and/or groups of workers that are considered high risk for experiencing adverse health effects related to occupational exposures. **If surveillance activities do detect an adverse health effect,** it is important that the appropriate control measures be instituted before the employees at risk are allowed to return to their job. It is also important that any workers at risk of exposure be placed under regular surveillance to confirm the success of control measures. If control measures are deemed ineffective, the employees at risk for exposure should be removed from the environment until the situation can be satisfactorily improved.

Role of Employee Cooperation and Participation

While these types of programs are an important part of an occupational health and safety program, they are not often mandated by the Occupational Safety and Health Administration (OSHA). Thus, **employee cooperation** is a critical element to the success of any health/medical surveillance program. For this reason, health education and promotion activities are important ways for the occupational health nurse to provide employees with the information they need to fully participate in the program.

Legal/Ethical Issues

American Association of Occupational Health Nurses' Code of Ethics

In order to address the issues within the field of nursing and to establish a standard for ethical conduct, the American Association of Occupational Health Nurses has established a **code of ethics** (AAOHN, 2016). The nine primary areas for ethical practice and behavior that make up this code of ethics are as follows:

1. The OHN articulates nursing values, maintains integrity of the profession, and integrates principles of social justice.
2. The OHN practices with compassion and respect for the dignity, worth, and unique attributes of every person.
3. The OHN's primary commitment is to the client, whether an individual, group, community, or population.
4. The OHN promotes, advocates for, and protects the rights, health, and safety of the client.
5. The OHN has authority, accountability, and responsibility for nursing practice; makes decisions; and takes action consistent with the obligation to prevent illness and injury, promote health, and provide optimal health care.
6. The OHN owes the same duties to self as to others by promoting health and safety, preserving wholeness of character and integrity, maintaining competence, and continuing personal and professional growth.
7. The OHN establishes, maintains, and improves the ethical environment of the work setting and conditions of employment that are conducive to safe and quality health care.
8. The OHN helps advance the nursing profession through research and scholarly inquiry, standards development and policy generation.
9. The OHN collaborates with other professionals to protect human rights, promote health, and reduce health disparities.

Legal Terms

Basic legal terms useful in occupational health are defined below:

- **Tort** – In civil law, a wrong committed against a person or their property. Examples include fraud, invasion of privacy, and defamation.
- **Nursing negligence** – Actions the compromise the standard of care to which all nurses are supposed to be committed.
- **Informed consent** – A patient must be educated and informed of the risks associated with procedure and have a thorough understanding of this before receiving treatment.
- **Malpractice** – Neglect of a patient that comes from unprofessional conduct or lack of skill.
- **Statute of limitations** – The time limit for filing a lawsuit after a wrong is committed. The statute of limitations for negligence is typically 2 years, and malpractice is 1 year.

Legal Responsibilities of Occupational Health Nurse

Within the field of occupational health nursing, there are **certain legal responsibilities** that a nurse must uphold. They are responsible for being up-to-date on any new or changed laws and regulations within their field. This includes changes from the State Board of Nursing, State Board of Pharmacy, and State Board of Medicine; as well as any changes in state and federal laws that could affect occupational health nursing. Furthermore, they must have an understanding of how actual nursing practice fits within the confines of these laws and regulations, as well as be capable of disputing regulations if deemed necessary.

OSHA

The **Occupational Safety and Health Act** (Public Law 91-596) became law in 1970 and was designed to ensure that every worker is allowed a safe and healthful work environment. This law excludes those that are self-employed, family farms that do not employ outside help, and industries regulated by other federal agencies. It was the OSH Act that prompted the creation of OSHA (Occupational Safety and Health Administration). OSHA carries out, administers, and enforces the health and safety standards established by the OSH Act. OSHA standards are legally enforceable and companies can be inspected for compliance at any time without advance notice. The OSH Act also created the National Institute for Occupational Safety and Health, which performs and funds occupational health and safety-related research programs.

Requirements for Recordkeeping

The **OSH Act (1970)** requires that most employers with more than 11 employees prepare and maintain records of work-related illnesses and injuries. The **OSHA 300 Log** is used to record this information. The types of illnesses and injuries that must be documented are those that result in death, missed days of work, job restrictions, loss of consciousness, serious injuries or illnesses that are diagnosed by a physician, or those that involve major medical treatment. Additionally, work-related needle sticks or cuts contaminated with another person's blood and blood borne pathogen exposures must be recorded. Illnesses or injuries where the worker requests that their name not be recorded on the log must also be reported.

Access to Employee Exposure and Medical Records

The **OSHA Access to Employee Exposure and Medical Records Standard** requires that the worker (or a designated representative) must have access to their occupational health and medical records. According to this standard, access must be provided free of charge and within 15 days of the request. If the worker requests copies, the employer must provide a way to provide them. It also requires that the worker sign a written consent before any health information is released that includes information about which records are being released, the purpose of the release, to whom they are being released, date of authorization, authorization time period, the authority by which records are being requested, and the identification of the employee. Although workers must be allowed access to medical records, they should not be allowed to leave with the originals.

ADA of 1990

The **Americans with Disabilities Act (ADA)** of 1990 deals with the accessibility of American society to those who have disabilities. One is considered disabled if they are officially diagnosed with a physical or mental condition that limits their ability to participate in life activities. Employers with more than 15 employees must adhere to the ADA. Under the ADA, employers are prohibited from inquiring about a disability during a job interview and, provided the individual is qualified, they cannot deny an individual a job because of their disability. Furthermore, persons with disabilities must be provided with reasonable accommodations to do a job. The Equal Employment Opportunity Commission (EEOC) is responsible for the enforcement and regulation of the ADA.

FMLA of 1993

The **Family Medical Leave Act (FMLA)** of 1993 allows workers to take up to 12 weeks of unpaid leave within a year without losing their job (or without demotion) for the following reasons: birth and care of a child; adoption or foster placement of a child; care of a parent, spouse, or child with a serious health condition; the worker's own inability to work due to a serious health condition. In order to be covered by the FMLA, the worker must fit two qualifying conditions. First, they must work for an employer that has at least 50 workers within a 75-mile radius. Second, the worker must have worked for the employer for 12 months for at least 1,250 hours. Under the FMLA, a worker has the right to return to the same (or equal) job after the leave. The worker has the responsibility, however, to provide the employer with at least a 30-day notice whenever possible.

HIPAA

The **Health Insurance Portability and Accountability Act (HIPAA)** of 1996 addresses health insurance plans and coverage issues that used to limit the insurability of workers. Because of HIPAA, exclusions for preexisting conditions are limited; workers cannot be denied coverage based on their current health status; and workers that lose group coverage are receive better access to individual coverage. Additionally, HIPAA's Privacy Rule protects the health information of patients by prohibiting "covered entities" (i.e. healthcare providers, healthcare clearinghouses, and health plans) to disclose any protected health information except as necessary (i.e. for treatment, payment, etc.) Protected health information (PHI) includes anything that identifies the patient or is associated with the patient's health, healthcare treatment, or healthcare payment. While in most instances an occupational health nurse is considered a "covered entity" and cannot disclose information, there are some plans that are not covered by HIPAA's Privacy Rule. Some of the plans not covered include disability benefit plans, worker's compensation, and work-life benefits (adoption assistance, tuition reimbursement, etc.).

Proper Documentation

As a part of the legal responsibilities within occupational health nursing, nurses are required to keep complete and accurate **documentation** of all activities and communications that occur within the program. There are several rules for proper documentation. In order for the information documented to be considered legal, it must be written with permanent black ink, dated, and signed. The worker's name must appear on each page of a medical record. Electronic documentation must have security in place so that it cannot be altered. All documentation must be clear and concise. Worker comments or questions must also be incorporated. The person responsible for the documentation must be clearly identified. Any errors should be fixed as soon as possible, with the original words still legible and the correction dated and explained.

Worker's Compensation System

The **worker's compensation system** was developed to reimburse workers for work-related injuries and illnesses. The benefits included in a worker's compensation program include income replacement when a worker is unable to work; support for the worker's dependents in the case of work-related death; hospital, medical, and funeral expenses; and in some cases, travel and parking expenses associated with work-related injury or illness. In most cases, the employer must provide worker's compensation benefits regardless of whether or not an accident was a result of employee neglect. It is important that the employee understands that if they accept worker's compensation benefits, they are no longer able to seek legal actions against the employer for their injuries.

Lockout/Tagout Procedures

Lockout/tagout is a safety procedure used to maintain a safe environment when equipment is being serviced or maintained. The general procedure entails putting the relevant equipment in an "off" or "safe" position, locking it in that position (lockout), and placing a tag on the equipment as a warning (tagout). Once the equipment has been serviced and it is verified by qualified personnel to be in safe working order, the lockout/tagout devices may be removed. It is critical that there is a clear, written lockout/tagout protocol in place. Only those personnel that are trained in lockout/tagout procedures may employ them. This keeps the procedure safe and well managed so that no one is unintentionally injured due to improper utilization of the procedure.

PRECEPTING

Precepting is an important element of employee training and is commonly used in the fields of medicine and nursing but has application to other areas of work as well. While mentoring may entail a long-term relationship, precepting is usually a time-limited arrangement related to a term of study, an orientation period, or a clinical rotation. Preceptors must balance responsibilities and ensure that they are able to provide adequate supervision and guidance to new employees on a daily basis. This may require coordinating schedules and planning carefully to ensure all responsibilities can be met. Preceptors help new employees to understand their impact on in the workplace by including the employee in all activities. Preceptors may engage in shared work as well as direct supervision in order to improve the employees' skills. Preceptors should be knowledgeable and skilled and should have some training regarding the responsibilities of precepting.

Information Management/Recordkeeping

Information Management

The term **information management** refers to the compilation, storage, accessibility, and organization of information. This is accomplished through the use of organizational skills and technological applications. There is a great deal of information that is collected within the field of occupational health nursing, and it is the responsibility of the nurse to effectively manage it. Nursing informatics was developed to deal with the need to manage information within the field of nursing. It is a combination of computer science, information science, and nursing science that work together to both manage and process nursing information.

Effective Health Information System

There are several characteristics of an **effective health information system.** First of all, any system must be adaptable enough to meet new requirements technological advancements, as well as compatible with other information management systems within the organization. It should also be easy to understand and use, cost effective, efficient, and capable of producing necessary reports, letters, etc. Because privacy laws protect health and medical information, it must have sufficient security measures in place. Finally, it must be designed in such a way so as to maintain the accuracy of the data, particularly in the event of a system failure.

Internet and Intranet

The **Internet** is a worldwide network of computers that allows for communication and the sharing of information on a large scale. **Intranets**, however, are private networks that belong to a company or organization that are in place to facilitate communication with a limited number of users, usually those within the organization. Both the Internet and intranets are useful to an occupational health nurse. Because the Internet typically contains current information from a variety of areas, it is particularly useful for staying up-to-date on topics pertaining to health and legal issues. It is also commonly used today as a means of communicating with other professionals, locating and purchasing equipment, and marketing goods and services to potential customers. Intranets, because they are organization-specific, allow for a much more efficient and organized means of management, but do not have much impact on the world outside of the organization.

Electronic Tools for Information Management

There are several **electronic tools and communications systems** available to the occupational health nurse for information management. This includes the Internet, company intranets, and office management programs such as word processing programs, spreadsheet programs, relational database systems, and presentation programs. Additionally, communication systems that include voice mail and electronic mail (e-mail), allow for quick and efficient communication with other workers and professionals. Regardless of whether any of these electronic tools are used alone or together in various combinations, they can produce an accurately and efficiently organized information management system.

Occupational Health Records

Occupational health records are governed by OSHA while clinical health records are governed by HIPAA because of privacy issues. However, if the occupational health record contains PHI and this information is transmitted electronically, it is subject to HIPAA regulations (45 CFR 160.103). OSHA requires that occupational health records be maintained separately from clinical health records either through the use of separate systems or through safeguards that allow access to only specific parts of the record so that people who are unauthorized are prevented from obtaining access. The occupational health record typically includes reports of medical evaluations (such as for work injuries), required immunization record, records of health status, exposure records, laboratory reports, consent forms, Workers' Compensation/insurance forms, accident/injury reports, consultant reports, substance abuse screening, and any other work-related health matters. The occupational healthcare provider is allowed to disclose information to the employer, the worker involved, the government, and other authorized third parties, but information released should meet the minimum necessary standard. Occupational health records must be retained for 30 years.

Recordkeeping

Recordkeeping by the occupational health nurse is governed by both federal and state legislation. OSHA requires injury and illness records although some types of businesses and those with fewer than 10 employees may have partial exemptions. The occupational nurse must record every fatality, injury, or illness that is related to work and is a new case (that is the individual involved has not preciously experienced the same type of injury or illness). Injuries and illnesses must be recorded on the OSHA 300 log and 301 incident report within 7 days of knowledge of the event. The logs and incident reports must be retained for 5 years. Occupational health records may be used in civil and legal actions and to determine employee benefits, so all entries must be complete, signed, and dated. The occupational health nurse must be aware of confidentiality, and personal health information must be kept separate from occupational exposure records to prevent unauthorized access to PHI.

Risk Communication

Risk communication is important to apprise workers of injury/illness risks, possible exposure to toxic substances or biological agents, injuries related to improper ergonomics, and work stress. Risk communication should be based on risk assessment and should be targeted to the appropriate workers. The overall goal is to reduce workplace fear and anxiety, to reduce accidental injuries, and to ensure the wellbeing of the workforce. Avenues and methods of risk communication in occupation health include:

- **Training**: May be conducted one-on-one or in groups, depending on the type of training needed.
- **Posters and warning signs**: Must be posted where workers can readily see and access them.
- **Brochures, FAQ sheets**: Should provide clear, easily understandable information in language appropriate for the target audience.
- **Internet**: Information may be presented online so that workers can access it at times convenient for them.
- **Meetings**: Review of issues may be discussed in departmental or routine meetings, providing ample time for questions and answers.

COHN-S Practice Test

1. The primary role of the occupational health nurse is to:

a. protect and promote workers' health.
b. reduce costs.
c. prevent workplace accidents.
d. meet regulatory requirements.

2. What is the best method for assessing a worker with work restrictions or limitations?

a. Direct observation.
b. Review of supervisor's assessment.
c. Review of worker self-assessment.
d. Review of worker productivity reports.

3. In cost analysis, which of the following represents conformance costs?

a. Costs related to errors, failures, or defects, including duplications of service and malpractice.
b. All costs (processes, services, equipment, time, material, staff) necessary to provide products or processes without error.
c. Costs related to preventing errors, such as monitoring and evaluation.
d. Costs that are shared, such as infrastructure costs.

4. Which of the following is a tool that provides a client's self-assessment of functional health and quality-of-life issues?

a. Health Status Survey (SF-36).
b. Patient Health Questionnaire (PHQ).
c. Post-Deployment Clinical Assessment Tool (PDCAT).
d. Barthel Index.

5. What type of screening is used to identify hearing threshold levels?

a. Tympanometry.
b. Evoked response audiometry.
c. Pure tone audiometry.
d. Otoscopy.

6. Which of the following is the first step in crisis intervention?

a. Devising a plan.
b. Assessing problem and triggering event.
c. Teaching coping mechanisms.
d. Evaluating resources.

7. Which pulmonary function test measures the total volume of air expelled in a specific period of time during repetitive maximal effort?

a. Forced vital capacity (FVC).
b. Forced expiratory volume, 1 second (FEV_1).
c. Forced expiratory flow, 200-1200 ($FEF_{200\text{-}1200}$).
d. Maximal voluntary ventilation (MVV).

8. Which of the following terms is the legal element of negligence that refers to a failure to carry out duties in accordance with accepted and usual standards of practice?

a. Duty.
b. Breach.
c. Causation.
d. Harm.

9. Which of the following may be included in job accommodation for an office worker with fine motor impairment?

a. Providing speech recognition program for computer access.
b. Modifying workstation to increase accessibility.
c. Providing stand/lean stools.
d. Providing rolling safety ladders.

10. Using real tasks or simulated work-related tasks and progressive exercises to strengthen and condition a person to return to work is an example of which of the following?

a. Job coaching.
b. Work adjustment.
c. Transitional employment.
d. Work hardening.

11. What is the correct elbow angle for an office worker when sitting in a chair and using a computer keyboard?

a. 45 degrees.
b. 60 degrees.
c. 90 degrees.
d. 120 degrees.

12. When determining the burden of proof for acts of negligence, how would risk management classify willfully providing inadequate care while disregarding the safety and security?

a. Negligent conduct.
b. Gross negligence.
c. Contributory negligence.
d. Comparative negligence.

13. Which of the following methods is used to determine monetary savings resulting from planned interventions?

a. Cost-benefit analysis.
b. Cost-effective analysis.
c. Efficacy study.
d. Cost-utility analysis.

14. When implementing a plan for risk management, what should be the primary concern in the statement of purpose?

a. Reduction in financial risk.
b. Worker safety.
c. Decreased liability.
d. Scope of program.

15. Which governmental agency is responsible for bloodborne pathogens standards?

a. CDC.
b. OSHA.
c. EPA.
d. FDA.

16. A worker with chronic back pain from a non-work-related injury has returned to work but is frequently late because of morning stiffness and pain and difficulty accessing public transportation. Which of the following should the occupational health nurse recommend initially?

a. Reduced working hours.
b. Reassignment to a different job.
c. Termination.
d. Flexible work schedule.

17. With the Continuous Quality Improvement (CQI) model, the focus of improvement is on which of the following?

a. Processes.
b. Staff.
c. Administrative personnel.
d. Clients.

18. The primary focus of Worker's Compensation is to:

a. prevent economic hardship.
b. return people to work.
c. contain costs.
d. promote worker's safety.

19. Under provisions of the Americans with Disabilities Act (ADA), which of the following is not a required accommodation?

a. Restructuring a job.
b. Modifying a work schedule.
c. Providing interpreters or readers.
d. Creating a new job.

20. A worker has been away from the job because of a short-term disability and has requested a return to work. Which of the following actions is the first step in this process?

a. Meet with administration to discuss the case.
b. Meet with the worker to discuss needs and options.
c. Review Americans with Disabilities Act (ADA) requirements.
d. Request the worker's medical records.

21. Under provisions of the Family and Medical Leave Act (FMLA), how many workweeks of leave in a 12-month period is a worker entitled to in order to care for his son, an Army service member, who was seriously injured in a bombing incident?

a. 10.
b. 12.
c. 26.
d. 48.

22. What is the primary reason for establishing guidelines for critical incident stress management (CISM) to deal with workplace violence or other traumatic events?

a. Reduce post-traumatic stress syndrome.
b. Meet regulatory requirements.
c. Reduce absenteeism.
d. Retain staff.

23. What type of routine health surveillance is indicated for workers exposed to nitric acid in the workplace?

a. Eyes only.
b. Lungs, eyes, and skin.
c. Blood pressure.
d. Hemoglobin and hematocrit.

24. A worker has suffered a splash of muriatic acid into the eyes. Which of the following immediate treatments is indicated?

a. Cover eyes and transport to ED.
b. Apply antibiotic ophthalmic ointment.
c. Apply artificial tears.
d. Irrigate eyes with copious amounts of water or normal saline.

25. When using a two-step PPD procedure to do skin testing for tuberculosis, the second step in the testing should be completed within one to three:

a. hours of first step.
b. days of first step.
c. weeks of first step.
d. months of first step.

26. In the hierarchy of controls for hazards, such as working with hazardous chemicals, which of the following is the most effective?

a. Substitution.
b. Administrative controls.
c. Elimination.
d. Personal protective equipment.

27. Which ethical principle is involved when a worker who is pregnant is reassigned from a job that involves contact with teratogenic substances to a different job?

a. Nonmaleficence.
b. Autonomy.
c. Beneficence.
d. Justice.

28. The occupational health nurse determines that adequate staffing for a workplace location requires 160 hours per week for 52 weeks during the year. How many fulltime equivalent (FTE) staff persons are required?

a. 2.
b. 4.
c. 8.
d. 16.

29. Which of the following questions is appropriate to ask an applicant during an interview?

a. "How many years ago did you finish college?"
b. "Can you arrange day care for your child during work hours?"
c. "Do you have any health problems?"
d. "Can you provide an example of how you have dealt with issues of diversity at work?"

30. The occupational health nurse notes that one department in an organization has experienced a marked increase in accidents over the previous two-month period. What should the OHN's initial action be?

a. Institute safety training for the department.
b. Complete a worker survey.
c. Evaluate all departmental changes.
d. Recommend increased supervision.

31. If the goal of an occupational safety program is to reduce injuries by 10%, using data from the previous year as baseline, which of the following is a direct supporting objective?

a. The OHN will investigate accidents/injuries within 24 hours.
b. The administration will establish a surveillance program to track injuries.
c. The OHN will conduct research into workplace injuries.
d. The administration will share information across departments.

32. When training first responders, the occupational health nurse should stress which of the following actions as the first that responders should carry out at a scene of injury?

a. Evaluating victim need.
b. Treating life-threatening injuries.
c. Assisting with transport of victims.
d. Determining environmental safety.

33. Using Knowles' principles of andragogy for adult learners, which of the following would likely be the best motivating factor to promote participation in a training program?

a. Increased job safety
b. Self-improvement
c. Certificate of achievement
d. Peer pressure

34. The occupational health nurse uses electronic health records (EHRs) for employees. Which type of data misuse occurs when the system allows a vendor to access private information?

a. Security breach.
b. Identity theft.
c. Unauthorized access.
d. Privacy violation.

35. When conducting an education or training needs assessment, which of the following is the first step the occupational health nurse should carry out?

a. Obtain management support.
b. Conduct a cost-benefit analysis.
c. Obtain funding.
d. Obtain data.

36. When conducting respirator fit tests, according to OSHA protocols, for how long should each test exercise, such as breathing and talking (with the exception of the grimace test), be conducted?

a. 15 seconds.
b. 30 seconds.
c. 45 seconds.
d. 60 seconds.

37. On which of the following should a successful stress management program focus?

a. Personal issues.
b. Organizational needs.
c. Working conditions.
d. Coping skills.

38. Which of the following roles is usually a time-limited arrangement related to a term of study, such as a semester, orientation period, or a clinical rotation?

a. Coaching.
b. Preceptoring.
c. Mentoring.
d. Supervising.

39. What is included in the appropriate personal protective equipment (PPE) for a construction worker operating electrical equipment, such as saws and nail guns?

a. Safety footwear.
b. Respirator.
c. Facemask.
d. Latex or synthetic latex gloves.

40. During a worksite walkthrough, the occupational health nurse observes an unsafe condition and immediately notifies the supervisor. What additional step is required regarding the unsafe condition?

a. Notifying the chief executive officer of the company of the unsafe condition.
b. Notifying the insurance carrier for the company that an unsafe condition exists.
c. Documenting the unsafe condition and noting the date by which it will be corrected.
d. Documenting that a worksite walkthrough was completed, indicating the date and time.

41. A workplace is placing an order for 200 office chairs. What is the primary concern of the occupational health nurse related to the chair characteristics?

a. Material.
b. Adjustability.
c. Structure.
d. Cost.

42. Which hazard control measure is the most important for an excavation site?

a. Physical barriers.
b. Signs.
c. Lighting.
d. Personal protective equipment.

43. Of the following work-related injury cases, the most appropriate for case management is a worker who:

a. fell and fractured his wrist.
b. developed contact dermatitis.
c. had a crush injury that caused a high-energy pelvic fracture.
d. suffered a severe cut to his finger in an accident with an electric saw.

44. Which of the following is most effective when instituting an organization-wide smoking ban?

a. Smoking cessation classes.
b. Reward system for smoking cessation.
c. Punitive system for violators.
d. 60-day advance notice.

45. What is most important for an occupational health nurse when conducting a safety inspection?

a. Assistance of a supervisor.
b. Notes taking during the inspection.
c. Lack of interruptions.
d. Utilization of a checklist.

46. For which of the following are Workmen's Compensation data most useful?

a. Tracking occupational illness.
b. Determining safety measures.
c. Estimating frequency of particular occupational injuries.
d. Reducing costs of work-related injuries.

47. When the occupational health nurse develops a case management plan for an individual, who should routinely receive copies of the plan?

a. The individual and the case manager.
b. All parties providing care.
c. The individual and all parties providing care.
d. The case manager only.

48. What complementary therapy may prove most useful to a worker who experiences anxiety-related headaches?

a. Acupuncture.
b. Visualization/relaxation.
c. Homeopathy.
d. Chiropractic treatment.

49. What type of rehabilitation program is likely most effective for a worker who recently experienced a severe work-related traumatic brain injury?

a. Acute inpatient rehabilitation facility.
b. Long-term care facility.
c. Behavior management program.
d. Day treatment center.

50. Which type of budget is used to pay for general expenses, such as salary, education, insurance, and maintenance?

a. Capital.
b. Operating.
c. Cash balance.
d. Master.

Answer Key and Explanations

1. A: While all of these are important, the primary role of the occupational health nurse is to protect and promote workers' health. The OHN must consider the effect that work has on health as well as the effect that poor health has on productivity with a focus on preventing ill health by ensuring safe working conditions and reducing the risk of toxic exposures, stress, and accidents; treating illness or injuries occurring in the workplace; and promoting good health practices, such as proper diet, exercise, and smoking cessation.

2. D: While all of these are important, productivity reports provide the most useful information regarding a worker's ability to carry out work functions because they provide objective information that is quantifiable. Extended direct observation can provide helpful information, but the OHN usually has limited time for observation, and short-term observation may not be adequate. The supervisor's assessment and the worker's self-assessment may provide biased information, depending on the supervisor's attitude toward the worker and the worker's attitude toward the job.

3. C: Conformance costs include those related to preventing errors, such as monitoring and evaluation. Nonconformance costs are those related to errors, failures, and defects. These may include adverse events (such as infections), poor access due to staff shortages or cancellations, lost time, duplications of service, and malpractice. Error-free costs are all those costs in terms of processes, services, equipment, time, materials, and staffing that are necessary to providing a product or process that is without error from the onset. Indirect costs are shared costs, such as infrastructure costs and the cost of custodial services.

4. A: Health Status Survey (SF-36 or SF-12) is a tool that provides a client's self-assessment of functional health and quality-of-life issues. Patient Health Questionnaire (PHQ) is used to screen patients and monitor conditions related to mental health disorders, such as depression, anxiety, and substance abuse. Post-Deployment Clinical Assessment Tool (PDCAT) is used to screen returning military for mental health and substance abuse problems related to deployment, including PTSD, depression, anxiety, and alcoholism. The Barthel Index assesses the functional ability of older adults in relation to activities of daily living.

5. C: Pure tone audiometry (PTA): Identifies hearing threshold levels by subjective response to pure tones to note the softest perceptible sound. Evoked response audiometry (ERA): Uses data from scalp electrodes to determine the electrical activity generated by exposure to sound. Tympanometry: Uses an instrument to check transmission of sound through the middle ear and is usually done in conjunction with PTA. Otoscopy: Uses an instrument to evaluate the outer ear for abnormalities.

6. B: The first step in crisis intervention is a thorough evaluation and assessment of the problem and the triggering event as well as assessment of risks, such as suicide. A plan should be devised in collaboration with the individual, taking resources into consideration. Steps in intervention include helping the individual to gain understanding about the cause of the crisis, encouraging the individual to freely express thoughts and feelings, teaching the individual different coping mechanisms and adaptive behaviors, and encouraging social interaction.

7. D: Maximal voluntary ventilation (MVV) is the total volume of air exhaled in a specified period of time (such as 12 seconds) during repetitive maximal effort. Forced vital capacity (FVC) measures the amount of air expelled in forced maximal expiration. Forced expiratory volume (FEV_1) is the amount of air expelled in a specified time, usually the first second of expiration (time in seconds indicate by subscript number). Forced expiratory flow (FEF $_{200-1200}$) is the mean FEF between 200-1200 mL of FVC.

8. B: Breach is the legal element of negligence that refers to a failure to carry out duties in accordance with accepted and usual standards of practice. Duty is a legal responsibility or obligation that relates to a relationship (such as parent to protect his/her child) or statute (such as the requirement for a CCM to report child abuse). Causation is the direct proof that a breach of duty resulted in harm. Harm is the injury that results from a breach of duty.

9. A: Because fine motor impairment interferes with a person's ability to use their hands, a job accommodation might include a speech recognition program for computer access as well as alternative methods to answer the phone and adaptive writing materials, ergonomic tools, page turners, grip devices, book holders, arm supports, and modified keyboards. Those with gross motor impairment may require modification in the workstation, stand/lean stools, rolling safety ladders, desktop lazy Susans, and carts to transport materials.

10. D: Work hardening is using real tasks or simulated work-related tasks and progressive exercises to strengthen and condition a person to return to the workplace. Work adjustment is assessing work behavior to determine behaviors that are appropriate and inappropriate and then providing support to increase appropriate behaviors and improve job skills. Transitional employment is the non-competitive employment placement utilized with job coaching. Job coaching is placing a person in a position and using a job specialist to train the employee to do specific job-related tasks and to learn the necessary interpersonal skills needed for the job.

11. C: When a person is sitting and working on a computer, the elbows should be bent at a 90-degree angle and wrists held straight. The seat of the chair should be adjusted so that the person's feet are flat on the floor (or on a foot stool if the person is short) and the knees also bent at a 90-degree angle. The chair should provide support in the lower back and the angle of the back of the chair to the seat should be 90 degrees.

12. B: Gross negligence. Negligence indicates that *proper care* has not been provided, based on established standards. *Reasonable care* uses rationale for decision-making in relation to providing care. Negligent conduct indicates that an individual failed to provide reasonable care or to protect/assist another, based on standards and expertise. Gross negligence is willfully providing inadequate care while disregarding the safety and security of another. Contributory negligence involves the injured party contributing to his/her own harm. Comparative negligence attempts to determine what percentage amount of negligence is attributed to each individual involved.

13. A: A cost-benefit analysis uses average cost of an event and the cost of intervention to demonstrate savings. A cost-effective analysis measures the effectiveness of an intervention rather than the monetary savings. Efficacy studies may compare a series of cost-benefit analyses to determine the intervention with the best cost-benefit. They may also be used for process or product evaluation. Cost-utility analysis (CUA) is essentially a subtype of cost-effective analysis, but it is more complex and the results are more difficult to quantify and use to justify expense because cost-utility analysis measures benefit to society in general, such as decreasing teen pregnancy.

14. B: Worker safety should always be the primary concern for risk management. Reduction of financial risks and liability relate directly to worker safety. A risk management plan should include:

- Goals: specific and measurable
- Program scope: should include linkage with other programs

- Line of authority: beginning with the governing board and ending with employees
- Policies: this should include confidentiality and conflict of interest
- Data sources and referrals: types of measures
- Documentation/reporting: the responsibility for reporting should be clarified and the frequency of reports
- Activities integration
- Evaluation of program: the method and frequency of evaluation
- Charts/diagrams: flow charts, organizational charts, and diagrams

15. B: OSHA, under the Department of Labor, is responsible for bloodborne pathogens standards as well as other workplace standards and inspection of workplaces to ensure safety standards are met. The CDC provides treatment guidelines and recommendations and monitors public health, compiling statistics regarding reportable disease. The EPA is not a statutory agency but provides information about the environment to other governmental agencies. The FDA is a consumer protection agency ensuring safety of medications, biological products, medical devices, and food.

16. D: Since arriving to work on time is the primary issue, allowing the worker a flexible work schedule will allow the person additional time in the morning when needed. Simply reducing hours or reassigning the worker may not solve the problem if the start-time remains the same, and these solutions may result in other problems, such as reduced pay or the need for retraining. Terminating a worker rather than offering reasonable accommodations may violate provisions of the ADA.

17. A: CQI emphasizes the organization, systems, and processes within that organization rather than individuals. It recognizes internal customers (staff) and external customers (clients) and utilizes data to improve processes, recognizing that most processes can be improved. CQI uses the scientific method of experimentation to meet needs and improve services and utilizes various tools, such as brainstorming, multivoting, various charts and diagrams, storyboarding, and meetings. Core concepts include:

- Quality and success is meeting or exceeding internal and external customers' needs and expectations.
- Problems relate to processes, and variations in process lead to variations in results.
- Change can be incremental.

18. B: The primary focus of Worker's Compensation, a type of insurance, is to return people to work as quickly and safely as possible. Worker's Compensation is intended for those who are injured on the job or whose health is impaired because of their jobs. Worker's Compensation provides 3 different types of benefits: cash to replace lost wages, reimbursement for medical costs associated with the injury, and death benefits to survivors. Worker's Compensation laws may vary somewhat from one state to another.

19. D: Employers must make reasonable accommodations for disabled workers but are not required to create a new job to meet the workers' needs. Most accommodations are usually relatively inexpensive for companies and can include reassigning a worker to a different open position, providing modified equipment (such as modified computers), allowing workers to sit rather than stand, preparing alternate training and examination materials, and providing a different workspace (such as one with fewer distractions or with easier access), and providing various assistive devices.

20. B: The first step in the process of returning a worker to work after a short-term disability is to meet with the worker to discuss the individual's needs and options to determine if the worker is able to return to work full-time or part-time and/or needs some other type of accommodations, such as a modified job or assignment to a different job in the company during a transition period. Armed with this information, the occupational health nurse can then decide what further steps to take.

21. C: FMLA allows 26 workweeks of leave in a 12-month period to provide care to a military service member who is a spouse, child, parent, or next-of-kin as part of military caregiver leave. Other entitlements include 12 workweeks of leave in a 12-month period for the birth of a child; adoption or foster care of a child (newly placed); illness of spouse, child, or parent; and a health condition that interferes with the ability to carry out job functions.

22. A: Critical incident stress management (CISM) helps workers cope with stressful events, such as workplace violence or disasters, in order to reduce incidence of post-traumatic stress syndrome. CISM includes a defusing session immediately after a stressful event followed by debriefing sessions in one to three days. The six phases of debriefing include introduction, fact sharing, discussing feelings, describing symptoms, teaching, and reentry. Follow-up is done at the end of the process, usually after about a week, but this can vary.

23. B: Workers exposed to nitric acid should have routine health surveillance for lungs, eyes, and skin. Nitric acid exposure may include ingestion, inhalation, or direct contact. Nitric acid may cause irritation and damage to the lungs, so periodic chest x-rays and pulmonary function tests are indicated. Nitric acid is also severely irritating to ocular tissue and may result in damage to the eyes. Prolonged contact with the skin may result in dermatitis. Workers with pre-existing disorders of the lungs, eyes, or skin are at increased risk.

24. D: Immediate treatment for chemical burns to the eyes includes irrigating the eyes and other areas of contact with copious amounts of water or normal saline. Many injuries are work-related and involve alkali (greater than 7 pH), acid (less than 7 pH) (muriatic acid or sulfuric acid), or other irritants (neutral pH), such as pepper spray. Alkali chemicals (such as ammonia, lime, and lye) usually cause the most serious injuries. Symptoms include pain, blurring of vision, tearing, and edema of eyelids.

25. C: A negative PPD finding can occur with an old infection because sensitivity wanes over time; however, subsequent tests months later might react positively because of the "booster phenomenon" caused by the first test. Therefore, a second test is done one to three weeks after the first to determine the effect of the first test. If the second test converts to positive in this short period of time, then it is considered evidence of a boosted reaction to a previous infection. If the second test is negative, it is considered a true negative and subsequent changes to positive would be considered new infections.

26. C: In the hierarchy of controls for hazards, elimination of the hazard is the most effective method of reducing risk, and this should be the goal when possible. Substitution, such as using a less hazardous chemical or procedure, provides the next best method followed by engineering controls (lifting devices, glove box, ventilation), administrative controls (alarms, labels, reduced duration of contact, and education), and the use of personal protective equipment (shields, gowns, gloves, safety glasses, ear plugs, hard hats).

27. A: Nonmaleficence is an ethical principle that means an employer should prevent intentional harm to the worker, such as by reassigning a pregnant worker to a job that does not endanger the fetus. Beneficence is the ethical principle that involves performing actions that are for the purpose of benefitting another person. Autonomy is the ethical principle that the individual has the right to make decisions about his/her own work. Justice is the ethical principle that relates to the distribution of the limited resources.

28. B: Four fulltime equivalent (FTE) staff persons are required. The formula for calculating fulltime equivalent (FTE) staffing helps to determine staffing needs:

- 40 hr/wk x 52 wk/yr = 1 FTE
- 160 hr/wk x 52 wk/yr = 4 FTE
- 20 hr/wk x 52 wk/yr = 0.5 FTE

Staffing must include coverage/policies for break and meal times. Staffing includes both daytime hours and nighttime. Workplaces vary in shift duration: five 8-hour shifts, four 10-hour shifts, or three 12-hour shifts, but overtime pay may be a consideration with longer shifts.

29. D: An appropriate interview question is "Can you provide an example of how you have dealt with issues of diversity at work?" because it relates to performance. The OHN should avoid asking questions that may be interpreted as age discrimination, such as questions about when a person finished college, or personal/family questions, such as about caring for children, because these are not job-related and may suggest bias. The OHN can ask applicants if they need work accommodations but not if they have health problems.

30. C: The initial action should be to evaluate all departmental changes that have occurred and may have resulted in more accidents. This may include new staff, changes in equipment, or different procedures. This information, coupled with data about the types of injuries, may help the OHN to focus on the cause of the problem and arrive at the best solution, which may include altering processes or changing equipment, instituting safety training, doing job-specific training, conducting surveys, providing assistive devices, or increasing supervision.

31. A: Objectives are the steps taken to achieve specific goals, so the OHN's investigating accidents and injuries within 24 hours provides the best means to determine the cause of the accidents/injuries and formulate preventive measures. Goals should be achievable aims, essentially end results, developed for specific units of the organization or the organization in general, focusing on improving performance. Objectives should be measurable and should include a timeline and identification of responsibility for achieving the objective.

32. D: The first action that first responders should carry out at a scene of injury is to determine environmental safety. That is, they should survey the area to determine that they can proceed safely to aid the victim without endangering themselves. Environmental concerns can include downed power lines, falling debris, flooding, explosives, toxic chemicals, or fire. In some cases, assailants, such as those with guns or knives, may pose a physical threat. If the first responders cannot proceed safely, they must wait for appropriate help, such as the police or fire department.

33. C: Adults are motivated by tangible rewards, such as certificates of achievement. Characteristics include:

Practical and goal-oriented	Provide overviews or summaries and examples. Use collaborative discussions with problem-solving exercises. Remain organized with the goal in mind.
Self-directed	Provide active involvement, asking for input. Allow different options toward achieving the goal. Give them responsibilities.
Knowledgeable	Show respect for their life experiences/ education. Validate their knowledge and ask for feedback. Relate new material to information with which they are familiar.
Relevancy-oriented	Explain how information will be applied. Clearly identify objectives.
Motivated	Provide certificates of achievement or some type of recognition for achievement.

34. A: Security breach: Careless or inadequate security allows others, such as billing companies or vendors, to have access to private information. Identity theft: Someone obtains identifying information, such as Social Security numbers, credit card numbers, birthdates, and addresses, for fraudulent purposes. Unauthorized access: Although EHRs and computerized documentation systems are password protected, providers sometimes share passwords or unwittingly expose their passwords to others when logging in, allowing others to access information about patients. Privacy violations: Even those authorized to access a patient's record may share private information with others, such as family or friends.

35. D: The first step in education and training needs assessment is to obtain data to help determine organizational, departmental, task, and individual training needs. Data may be obtained from surveys, interviews, observations, focus groups, review of documents, and advisory groups. Once needs are determined, then the OHN should determine the type of training needed and the steps needed to develop a training program. Additionally, the OHN should conduct a cost-benefit analysis in order to obtain management support and funding.

36. D: Each test exercise for respirator fit should be conducted for 60 seconds except for the grimace test, which is conducted for 15 seconds. Test exercises include normal and deep breathing, moving the head up and down and side to side, talking (reading or reciting), and bending over at the waist (or jogging in place if the respirator prevents this action). Additionally, odor threshold screening and testing are conducted. Tests cannot be conducted where there is hair, such as a beard, between skin and sealing surface.

37. C: While personal issues, such as an individual's response to stress, are important along with coping skills, the primary cause of stress in the workplace is workplace demands, such as unrealistic workloads or deadlines and unclear job descriptions, so the primary focus should be on improving the working conditions that result in stress. Surveys about job satisfaction and workplace concerns may be a good starting point because encouraging workers to express concerns is one method of reducing stress.

38. B: Preceptoring is usually a time-limited arrangement related to a term of study, such as a semester, orientation period, or a clinical rotation. The preceptor may engage in shared care as well as direct supervision to improve the student's skills. Mentoring usually involves an experienced professional providing support and encouragement to someone with less experience in an ongoing relationship. Coaching is a component of both mentoring and preceptoring and includes giving positive feedback, questioning, providing demonstrations, providing progress reports, assisting students to establish improvement goals, and providing resources. Supervising involves monitoring work activities.

39. A: PPE for construction workers includes safety footwear, such as steel-toe boots; safety glasses to protect the eyes from intense light, dust, and fragments of wood or other materials; a hard hat to protect the head from falling materials; safety gloves, such as welders' gloves or cut-resistant gloves, to protect the hands; ear protection, such as earplugs; and fall protection equipment for those working at a height, such as on a roof or in a high-rise building.

40. C: When the OHN finds an unsafe condition during a worksite walkthrough, the OHN must document the unsafe condition in detail as part of the report, indicating the date by which the unsafe condition will be corrected. Aside from that, notifications depend on the company structure (size and hierarchy) and the severity of the unsafe condition. All worksite walkthroughs must be documented to show date and time and records kept to demonstrate that routine inspections have been done.

41. B: Adjustability is the primary concern related to the office chairs because chairs must be adjusted for individuals in order to maintain proper body alignment and support. Chairs should provide arm and lumbar support. Additionally, pan length may vary or should be ordered in different sizes to accommodate small or large adults. Some chairs should be purchased in extra wide widths to accommodate overweight individuals. Ideally, chairs should recline to relieve back strain, especially for workers who spend hours in their chairs.

42. A: While all of these are important as hazard control measures, the most important is to ensure that a physical barrier, such as fencing, is in place to prevent unauthorized access to the site. There should be adequate warning signs that are easily seen and in large type placed on all accessible sides of the excavation site. Workers in the excavation area should wear appropriate PPE, and working conditions and ground stability should be monitored carefully.

43. C: All of these injuries have a relatively predictable course of recovery except for the crush injury that caused a high-energy pelvic fracture, so this worker should receive case management services. High-energy fractures may result in internal organ damage as well as hemorrhage, and the worker may be out of work for months during the recovery process and may require a number of different rehabilitative services as well as work accommodations when returning to the workforce.

44. A: Smoking cessation classes are the most effective measures to promote cooperation when instituting an organization-wide smoking ban because classes provide tools for those who are willing to quit. Punitive systems cause resentment while reward systems may encourage people to stop smoking, but without the support of classes, many will resume smoking within a short period. Smokers should have a plan that sets a date (within 2 weeks), removes cigarettes, enlists family and friends, reviews past attempts, and anticipates challenges during the withdrawal period.

45. D: The occupational health nurse should always use a detailed checklist when conducting a safety inspection because each area of an organization may have very different safety concerns. The entire work area should be carefully inspected in an organized sequence, following the checklist in order. A supervisor or knowledgeable worker should also be available during the inspection to answer questions, and the OHN should question workers as necessary to clarify concerns about safety issues. All safety violations and hazardous conditions must be carefully documented.

46. C: Workman's Compensation data are not available on a national basis and criteria for data collection may vary from state to state along with state regulations. Even limited (statewide) data may provide an estimate of the occupational injuries as well as associated costs. The data may help guide the institution of work safety measures and development of safety training. Occupational illness data are less useful because injuries tend to be similar across industries, whereas illnesses show more variation.

47. A: The individual for whom the case management plan is created and the case manager should both routinely have copies of the plan. All parties providing care may, with permission of the individual, receive a copy of the case management plan if it will aid in meeting the individual's care needs. Because of privacy concerns, the case management plan cannot be widely distributed because the services provided may divulge information about the individual's diagnosis and treatment.

48. B: Visualization/relaxation is creating a visual image in the mind of a desired outcome and imagining or "feeling" oneself in that place or situation. Intense concentration helps to block feelings of anxiety. For example, if the focus is on reducing anxiety, the mind focuses on that goal of therapy. All of the senses may be used to imagine the feeling of being in a place and feeling very relaxed—what it looks like, smells like, feels like, and sounds like.

49. A: A worker who experienced a recent severe traumatic brain injury would probably benefit most from an acute inpatient rehabilitation facility so that the worker can receive intensive specialized assessment and treatment. Behavior management programs are usually outpatient facilities that teach people to exercise self-control and to behave in a socially acceptable manner. Long-term care facilities are for those who have are unable to live alone despite therapy. Day-treatment programs provide therapy for those with lesser injuries who are able to return home after treatment.

50. B: Operating budget: Used for daily operations and includes general expenses, such as salaries, education, insurance, maintenance, depreciation, debts, and profit. The budget has 3 elements: statistics, expenses, and revenue. Capital budget: Determines which capital projects (such as remodeling, repairing, and purchasing of equipment or buildings) will be allocated funding for the year. These capital expenditures are usually based on cost-benefit analysis and prioritization of needs. Cash balance budget: Projects cash balances for a specific future time period, including all operating and capital budget items. Master budget: Combines operating, capital and cash balance budgets as well as any specialized or area-specific budgets.

How to Overcome Test Anxiety

Just the thought of taking a test is enough to make most people a little nervous. A test is an important event that can have a long-term impact on your future, so it's important to take it seriously and it's natural to feel anxious about performing well. But just because anxiety is normal, that doesn't mean that it's helpful in test taking, or that you should simply accept it as part of your life. Anxiety can have a variety of effects. These effects can be mild, like making you feel slightly nervous, or severe, like blocking your ability to focus or remember even a simple detail.

If you experience test anxiety—whether severe or mild—it's important to know how to beat it. To discover this, first you need to understand what causes test anxiety.

Causes of Test Anxiety

While we often think of anxiety as an uncontrollable emotional state, it can actually be caused by simple, practical things. One of the most common causes of test anxiety is that a person does not feel adequately prepared for their test. This feeling can be the result of many different issues such as poor study habits or lack of organization, but the most common culprit is time management. Starting to study too late, failing to organize your study time to cover all of the material, or being distracted while you study will mean that you're not well prepared for the test. This may lead to cramming the night before, which will cause you to be physically and mentally exhausted for the test. Poor time management also contributes to feelings of stress, fear, and hopelessness as you realize you are not well prepared but don't know what to do about it.

Other times, test anxiety is not related to your preparation for the test but comes from unresolved fear. This may be a past failure on a test, or poor performance on tests in general. It may come from comparing yourself to others who seem to be performing better or from the stress of living up to expectations. Anxiety may be driven by fears of the future—how failure on this test would affect your educational and career goals. These fears are often completely irrational, but they can still negatively impact your test performance.

Review Video: 3 Reasons You Have Test Anxiety
Visit mometrix.com/academy and enter code: 428468

Elements of Test Anxiety

As mentioned earlier, test anxiety is considered to be an emotional state, but it has physical and mental components as well. Sometimes you may not even realize that you are suffering from test anxiety until you notice the physical symptoms. These can include trembling hands, rapid heartbeat, sweating, nausea, and tense muscles. Extreme anxiety may lead to fainting or vomiting. Obviously, any of these symptoms can have a negative impact on testing. It is important to recognize them as soon as they begin to occur so that you can address the problem before it damages your performance.

Review Video: 3 Ways to Tell You Have Test Anxiety
Visit mometrix.com/academy and enter code: 927847

The mental components of test anxiety include trouble focusing and inability to remember learned information. During a test, your mind is on high alert, which can help you recall information and stay focused for an extended period of time. However, anxiety interferes with your mind's natural processes, causing you to blank out, even on the questions you know well. The strain of testing during anxiety makes it difficult to stay focused, especially on a test that may take several hours. Extreme anxiety can take a huge mental toll, making it difficult not only to recall test information but even to understand the test questions or pull your thoughts together.

Review Video: How Test Anxiety Affects Memory
Visit mometrix.com/academy and enter code: 609003

Effects of Test Anxiety

Test anxiety is like a disease—if left untreated, it will get progressively worse. Anxiety leads to poor performance, and this reinforces the feelings of fear and failure, which in turn lead to poor performances on subsequent tests. It can grow from a mild nervousness to a crippling condition. If allowed to progress, test anxiety can have a big impact on your schooling, and consequently on your future.

Test anxiety can spread to other parts of your life. Anxiety on tests can become anxiety in any stressful situation, and blanking on a test can turn into panicking in a job situation. But fortunately, you don't have to let anxiety rule your testing and determine your grades. There are a number of relatively simple steps you can take to move past anxiety and function normally on a test and in the rest of life.

Review Video: How Test Anxiety Impacts Your Grades
Visit mometrix.com/academy and enter code: 939819

Physical Steps for Beating Test Anxiety

While test anxiety is a serious problem, the good news is that it can be overcome. It doesn't have to control your ability to think and remember information. While it may take time, you can begin taking steps today to beat anxiety.

Just as your first hint that you may be struggling with anxiety comes from the physical symptoms, the first step to treating it is also physical. Rest is crucial for having a clear, strong mind. If you are tired, it is much easier to give in to anxiety. But if you establish good sleep habits, your body and mind will be ready to perform optimally, without the strain of exhaustion. Additionally, sleeping well helps you to retain information better, so you're more likely to recall the answers when you see the test questions.

Getting good sleep means more than going to bed on time. It's important to allow your brain time to relax. Take study breaks from time to time so it doesn't get overworked, and don't study right before bed. Take time to rest your mind before trying to rest your body, or you may find it difficult to fall asleep.

Review Video: The Importance of Sleep for Your Brain
Visit mometrix.com/academy and enter code: 319338

Along with sleep, other aspects of physical health are important in preparing for a test. Good nutrition is vital for good brain function. Sugary foods and drinks may give a burst of energy but this burst is followed by a crash, both physically and emotionally. Instead, fuel your body with protein and vitamin-rich foods.

Also, drink plenty of water. Dehydration can lead to headaches and exhaustion, especially if your brain is already under stress from the rigors of the test. Particularly if your test is a long one, drink water during the breaks. And if possible, take an energy-boosting snack to eat between sections.

Review Video: How Diet Can Affect your Mood
Visit mometrix.com/academy and enter code: 624317

Along with sleep and diet, a third important part of physical health is exercise. Maintaining a steady workout schedule is helpful, but even taking 5-minute study breaks to walk can help get your blood pumping faster and clear your head. Exercise also releases endorphins, which contribute to a positive feeling and can help combat test anxiety.

When you nurture your physical health, you are also contributing to your mental health. If your body is healthy, your mind is much more likely to be healthy as well. So take time to rest, nourish your body with healthy food and water, and get moving as much as possible. Taking these physical steps will make you stronger and more able to take the mental steps necessary to overcome test anxiety.

Review Video: How to Stay Healthy and Prevent Test Anxiety
Visit mometrix.com/academy and enter code: 877894

Mental Steps for Beating Test Anxiety

Working on the mental side of test anxiety can be more challenging, but as with the physical side, there are clear steps you can take to overcome it. As mentioned earlier, test anxiety often stems from lack of preparation, so the obvious solution is to prepare for the test. Effective studying may be the most important weapon you have for beating test anxiety, but you can and should employ several other mental tools to combat fear.

First, boost your confidence by reminding yourself of past success—tests or projects that you aced. If you're putting as much effort into preparing for this test as you did for those, there's no reason you should expect to fail here. Work hard to prepare; then trust your preparation.

Second, surround yourself with encouraging people. It can be helpful to find a study group, but be sure that the people you're around will encourage a positive attitude. If you spend time with others who are anxious or cynical, this will only contribute to your own anxiety. Look for others who are motivated to study hard from a desire to succeed, not from a fear of failure.

Third, reward yourself. A test is physically and mentally tiring, even without anxiety, and it can be helpful to have something to look forward to. Plan an activity following the test, regardless of the outcome, such as going to a movie or getting ice cream.

When you are taking the test, if you find yourself beginning to feel anxious, remind yourself that you know the material. Visualize successfully completing the test. Then take a few deep, relaxing breaths and return to it. Work through the questions carefully but with confidence, knowing that you are capable of succeeding.

Developing a healthy mental approach to test taking will also aid in other areas of life. Test anxiety affects more than just the actual test—it can be damaging to your mental health and even contribute to depression. It's important to beat test anxiety before it becomes a problem for more than testing.

Review Video: Test Anxiety and Depression
Visit mometrix.com/academy and enter code: 904704

Study Strategy

Being prepared for the test is necessary to combat anxiety, but what does being prepared look like? You may study for hours on end and still not feel prepared. What you need is a strategy for test prep. The next few pages outline our recommended steps to help you plan out and conquer the challenge of preparation.

Step 1: Scope Out the Test

Learn everything you can about the format (multiple choice, essay, etc.) and what will be on the test. Gather any study materials, course outlines, or sample exams that may be available. Not only will this help you to prepare, but knowing what to expect can help to alleviate test anxiety.

Step 2: Map Out the Material

Look through the textbook or study guide and make note of how many chapters or sections it has. Then divide these over the time you have. For example, if a book has 15 chapters and you have five days to study, you need to cover three chapters each day. Even better, if you have the time, leave an extra day at the end for overall review after you have gone through the material in depth.

If time is limited, you may need to prioritize the material. Look through it and make note of which sections you think you already have a good grasp on, and which need review. While you are studying, skim quickly through the familiar sections and take more time on the challenging parts. Write out your plan so you don't get lost as you go. Having a written plan also helps you feel more in control of the study, so anxiety is less likely to arise from feeling overwhelmed at the amount to cover.

Step 3: Gather Your Tools

Decide what study method works best for you. Do you prefer to highlight in the book as you study and then go back over the highlighted portions? Or do you type out notes of the important information? Or is it helpful to make flashcards that you can carry with you? Assemble the pens, index cards, highlighters, post-it notes, and any other materials you may need so you won't be distracted by getting up to find things while you study.

If you're having a hard time retaining the information or organizing your notes, experiment with different methods. For example, try color-coding by subject with colored pens, highlighters, or post-it notes. If you learn better by hearing, try recording yourself reading your notes so you can listen while in the car, working out, or simply sitting at your desk. Ask a friend to quiz you from your flashcards, or try teaching someone the material to solidify it in your mind.

Step 4: Create Your Environment

It's important to avoid distractions while you study. This includes both the obvious distractions like visitors and the subtle distractions like an uncomfortable chair (or a too-comfortable couch that makes you want to fall asleep). Set up the best study environment possible: good lighting and a comfortable work area. If background music helps you focus, you may want to turn it on, but otherwise keep the room quiet. If you are using a computer to take notes, be sure you don't have any other windows open, especially applications like social media, games, or anything else that could distract you. Silence your phone and turn off notifications. Be sure to keep water close by so you stay hydrated while you study (but avoid unhealthy drinks and snacks).

Also, take into account the best time of day to study. Are you freshest first thing in the morning? Try to set aside some time then to work through the material. Is your mind clearer in the afternoon or evening? Schedule your study session then. Another method is to study at the same time of day that you will take the test, so that your brain gets used to working on the material at that time and will be ready to focus at test time.

Step 5: Study!

Once you have done all the study preparation, it's time to settle into the actual studying. Sit down, take a few moments to settle your mind so you can focus, and begin to follow your study plan. Don't give in to distractions or let yourself procrastinate. This is your time to prepare so you'll be ready to fearlessly approach the test. Make the most of the time and stay focused.

Of course, you don't want to burn out. If you study too long you may find that you're not retaining the information very well. Take regular study breaks. For example, taking five minutes out of every hour to walk briskly, breathing deeply and swinging your arms, can help your mind stay fresh.

As you get to the end of each chapter or section, it's a good idea to do a quick review. Remind yourself of what you learned and work on any difficult parts. When you feel that you've mastered the material, move on to the next part. At the end of your study session, briefly skim through your notes again.

But while review is helpful, cramming last minute is NOT. If at all possible, work ahead so that you won't need to fit all your study into the last day. Cramming overloads your brain with more information than it can process and retain, and your tired mind may struggle to recall even previously learned information when it is overwhelmed with last-minute study. Also, the urgent nature of cramming and the stress placed on your brain contribute to anxiety. You'll be more likely to go to the test feeling unprepared and having trouble thinking clearly.

So don't cram, and don't stay up late before the test, even just to review your notes at a leisurely pace. Your brain needs rest more than it needs to go over the information again. In fact, plan to finish your studies by noon or early afternoon the day before the test. Give your brain the rest of the day to relax or focus on other things, and get a good night's sleep. Then you will be fresh for the test and better able to recall what you've studied.

Step 6: Take a practice test

Many courses offer sample tests, either online or in the study materials. This is an excellent resource to check whether you have mastered the material, as well as to prepare for the test format and environment.

Check the test format ahead of time: the number of questions, the type (multiple choice, free response, etc.), and the time limit. Then create a plan for working through them. For example, if you have 30 minutes to take a 60-question test, your limit is 30 seconds per question. Spend less time on the questions you know well so that you can take more time on the difficult ones.

If you have time to take several practice tests, take the first one open book, with no time limit. Work through the questions at your own pace and make sure you fully understand them. Gradually work up to taking a test under test conditions: sit at a desk with all study materials put away and set a timer. Pace yourself to make sure you finish the test with time to spare and go back to check your answers if you have time.

After each test, check your answers. On the questions you missed, be sure you understand why you missed them. Did you misread the question (tests can use tricky wording)? Did you forget the information? Or was it something you hadn't learned? Go back and study any shaky areas that the practice tests reveal.

Taking these tests not only helps with your grade, but also aids in combating test anxiety. If you're already used to the test conditions, you're less likely to worry about it, and working through tests until you're scoring well gives you a confidence boost. Go through the practice tests until you feel comfortable, and then you can go into the test knowing that you're ready for it.

Test Tips

On test day, you should be confident, knowing that you've prepared well and are ready to answer the questions. But aside from preparation, there are several test day strategies you can employ to maximize your performance.

First, as stated before, get a good night's sleep the night before the test (and for several nights before that, if possible). Go into the test with a fresh, alert mind rather than staying up late to study.

Try not to change too much about your normal routine on the day of the test. It's important to eat a nutritious breakfast, but if you normally don't eat breakfast at all, consider eating just a protein bar. If you're a coffee drinker, go ahead and have your normal coffee. Just make sure you time it so that the caffeine doesn't wear off right in the middle of your test. Avoid sugary beverages, and drink enough water to stay hydrated but not so much that you need a restroom break 10 minutes into the test. If your test isn't first thing in the morning, consider going for a walk or doing a light workout before the test to get your blood flowing.

Allow yourself enough time to get ready, and leave for the test with plenty of time to spare so you won't have the anxiety of scrambling to arrive in time. Another reason to be early is to select a good seat. It's helpful to sit away from doors and windows, which can be distracting. Find a good seat, get out your supplies, and settle your mind before the test begins.

When the test begins, start by going over the instructions carefully, even if you already know what to expect. Make sure you avoid any careless mistakes by following the directions.

Then begin working through the questions, pacing yourself as you've practiced. If you're not sure on an answer, don't spend too much time on it, and don't let it shake your confidence. Either skip it and come back later, or eliminate as many wrong answers as possible and guess among the remaining ones. Don't dwell on these questions as you continue—put them out of your mind and focus on what lies ahead.

Be sure to read all of the answer choices, even if you're sure the first one is the right answer. Sometimes you'll find a better one if you keep reading. But don't second-guess yourself if you do immediately know the answer. Your gut instinct is usually right. Don't let test anxiety rob you of the information you know.

If you have time at the end of the test (and if the test format allows), go back and review your answers. Be cautious about changing any, since your first instinct tends to be correct, but make sure you didn't misread any of the questions or accidentally mark the wrong answer choice. Look over any you skipped and make an educated guess.

At the end, leave the test feeling confident. You've done your best, so don't waste time worrying about your performance or wishing you could change anything. Instead, celebrate the successful completion of this test. And finally, use this test to learn how to deal with anxiety even better next time.

Review Video: 5 Tips to Beat Test Anxiety
Visit mometrix.com/academy and enter code: 570656

Important Qualification

Not all anxiety is created equal. If your test anxiety is causing major issues in your life beyond the classroom or testing center, or if you are experiencing troubling physical symptoms related to your anxiety, it may be a sign of a serious physiological or psychological condition. If this sounds like your situation, we strongly encourage you to seek professional help.

Thank You

We at Mometrix would like to extend our heartfelt thanks to you, our friend and patron, for allowing us to play a part in your journey. It is a privilege to serve people from all walks of life who are unified in their commitment to building the best future they can for themselves.

The preparation you devote to these important testing milestones may be the most valuable educational opportunity you have for making a real difference in your life. We encourage you to put your heart into it—that feeling of succeeding, overcoming, and yes, conquering will be well worth the hours you've invested.

We want to hear your story, your struggles and your successes, and if you see any opportunities for us to improve our materials so we can help others even more effectively in the future, please share that with us as well. **The team at Mometrix would be absolutely thrilled to hear from you!** So please, send us an email (support@mometrix.com) and let's stay in touch.

If you'd like some additional help, check out these other resources we offer for your exam: http://mometrixflashcards.com/COHN

Additional Bonus Material

Due to our efforts to try to keep this book to a manageable length, we've created a link that will give you access to all of your additional bonus material.

Please visit https://www.mometrix.com/bonus948/cohns to access the information.